Introduction

This book is particularly useful when used with the *A to Z of Peripheral Nerves* and the *A to Z of the Bones, Joints, Ligaments & the Back*, The *A to Z of Skeletal Muscles* and the *A to Z of the Brain and Cranial Nerves* but all the A to Zs are cross-referenced and together are forming a set covering the all structural elements of the human body; and now including pathological considerations in the new ***The A to Z of... failure*** series e.g. The *A to Z of Bone & Joint Failure.*

If there is a structure/subject you want to see in the A to Zs let us know.

The A to Zs may be viewed on 2 sites – www.amandasatoz.com and http://www.aspenpharma.com.au/atlas/student.htm

Acknowledgement

I would like to thank Aspenpharmacare Australia: Mr Greg Lan CEO, & Mr Robert Koster in particular & all those who have helped in the contribution of this edition & in the feedback of the other books in this series. Thankyou.

Dedication To hard work but not necessarily to working hard.

How to use this book

The format of this A to Z book has been maintained as in the last edition - the bones of the Head & Neck are in the front followed by the muscles. Each section listed in alphabetical order as with the other A to Zs. The book is its own index in each section. In the front of each section, as usual, there are overviews of bone or muscle groupings such as the bones surrounding and forming cranial cavities and groupings of muscles around the larynx, as well as individual views of each and every bone and muscle. The skull has a separate listing.

As with all the A to Zs - think of it and then find it alphabetically. Cross referencing in the index is in the usual manner i.e. see for go to and see also for additional images listed under that heading.

Thank you,

A. L. Neill
BSc MSc MBBS PhD FACBS
medicalamanda@gmail.com
ISBN 978-1-921930-12-6

T0329505

© A. L. Neill

Table of contents

Abbreviations

A	= actions / movements of a joint		jt(s)	= joints = articulations
aa	= anastomosis or anastomoses		L	= lumbar / left
ACF	= anterior cranial fossa		LL	= lower limb
adj.	= adjective		lig	= ligament
aka	= also known as		LP	= lumbar plexus
ALL	= anterior longitudinal ligament		Lt.	= Latin
alt.	= alternative		MCF	= middle cranial fossa
ANS	= autonomic nervous system		MCL	= mid clavicular line
ant.	= anterior		med	= medial
art.	= articulation (joint w/o the additional support structures)		mm	= mucous membranes
AS	= Alternative Spelling, generally referring to the diff. b/n British & American spelling		N (s)	= nerve(s)
			NAD	= normal (size, shape)
			NAD	= no abnormality detected
			NR	= nerve root origin
ASIS	= anterior superior iliac spine (of hip bone)		NS	= nervous supply / nerve system
			NT	= nervous tissue
bc	= because		nv	= neurovascular bundle
b/n	= between		O	= origin
BP	= brachial plexus		P	= pressure
BS	= Blood Supply		PaNS.	= parasympathetic nervous system
BVs	= blood vessels		ParaNs	= parasympathetic nerves ± fibres
C	= cervical		pl.	= plural
c.f.	= compared to		PLL	= posterior longitudinal ligament
CF	= cranial fossa		PM	= pia mater
CH	= cerebral hemispheres		PN	= peripheral nerve
CN	= cranial nerve		post.	= posterior
CNS	= central nervous system		proc.	= process
Co	= coccygeal		prox.	= proximal
CP	= cervical plexus		R	= right / resistance
collat.	= collateral		ROM	= range of motion
Cr	= cranial		sing.	= singular
CSF	= Cerebrospinal fluid		SC	= spinal cord
CT	= connective tissue		SN	= spinal nerve
diff.	= difference(s)		SP	= spinous process / sacral plexus
dist.	= distal		SS	= signs and symptoms
DM	= dura mater		supf	= superficial
EB	= eyeball		T	= TEST / thoracic
e.g.	= example		TOS	= thoracic outlet syndrome
EAM	= external acoustic meatus		T	= transverse process
EC	= extracellular (outside the cell)		UL	= upper limb, arm
EOM	= extra-ocular muscles		VB	= vertebral body
ES	= Erector Spinae group of muscles		VC	= vertebral column
ext.	= extensor (as in muscle to extend across a joint)		WM	= white matter
			w/n	= within
Gk.	= Greek		w/o	= without
GM	= Grey matter		wrt	= with respect to
I	= insertion		&	= and
IAM	= internal acoustic meatus			= intersection with
IOM	= intra-ocular muscles			

Ablation   The removal of part of the body, generally a bony part, most commonly the teeth.

Acral   in the extremities - bones at the apex or end of limbs

Acromegaly   A continuation of growth of the ends of cartilage covered bone (after fusion of the long bones) hence a gross change in the features (most noticeable in the jaw and digits) without growth in height, due mainly to the over activity of the pituitary gland.

Ala   A wing, hence a wing-like process as in the Ethmoid bone *pl. - alae.*

Alveolus   Air filled bone - tooth socket *adj. - alveolar* (as in air filled bone in the maxilla) - coalescence of alveoli helps in the formation of the sinuses. This device also lightens the weight of the bone particularly the skull.

Ankle   Bend = angle usually referring to the bend just above the foot, hence the ankle is the joint b/n the foot and the lower leg.

Annulus fibrosis   The peripheral fibrous ring around the intervertebral disc.

Aperture   An opening or space between bones or within a bone.

Appendicular   Refers to the appendices of the axial i.e. in the skeleton, the limbs upper and lower which hang from the axial skeleton, this also includes the pectoral and pelvic girdles but not the sacrum.

Areola   Small, open spaces as in the areolar part of the Maxilla may lead or develop into sinuses.

Arth-   To do with joints hence…
Arthritis   Inflammation of a joint.

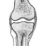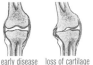

early disease   loss of cartilage   inflammation of jt   laxity of lig & permanent damage

Arthropathy   Diseases of the joints.
Arthrosis   Joint types.
Articulation   Joint, description of the bone surfaces joining w/o the supporting structures = point of contact b/n 2 opposing bones hence the articulation of humerus and scapula is the articulation of the shoulder joint.

Attrition   Tooth wear and tear.

Auditory   Pertaining to hearing, hence, pertaining to the ear. (*Auditory exostosis* = a bony growth on the walls of the External Auditory Meatus).

Avulsion   Forceable tearing away of a structure or part of a structure as in an avulsed fracture where a fragment bone is torn away from the main bone.

Axial   Refers to the head and trunk (vertebrae, ribs & sternum) of the body.

Ball and Socket   Generally referring to a joint which resembles a ball sitting tightly in a socket - very stable, limited range of movement e.g. hip joint.

Basilar   Relating to the base or bottom of structures.

Basiocranium   Bones of the base of the skull.

Boss   A smooth round broad eminence - mainly in the frontal bone female > male.

Bregma   Refers to a junction of more than 2 bones in a joint as in the Bregma of the skull, junction between the coronal and sagittal sutures which in the infant is not closed and can be felt pulsating - site of the anterior fontanelle.

Buccal   Pertaining to the cheek.

Callus	Hard tissue formed in the osteogenic layer of the periosteum as a fracture repair tissue it is replaced over time with compact bone.
Calotte	The calotte consists of the calvaria from which the base has been removed
Calvaria	The calvaria refers to the cranium without the facial bones attached.
Canal	Tunnel / extended foramen as in the carotid canal at the base of the skull *adj.- canular* (canicular - small canal).
Cancellous bone	= Trabecular bone
	A spongy porous bone with spicules (trabeculae) of compact bone. It is found at the ends of long bones in the bones of the axial skeleton. Red BM is found b/n the spicules.
Caput / Kaput	The head or of a head, *adj.- capitate = having a head (c.f. decapitate)*
Carotid	To put to sleep; compression of the common or internal carotid artery causes coma. This refers to bony points related to the Carotid vessels.
Carpo	Wrist.
Cavity	An open area or sinus within a bone or formed by two or more bones *(adj.- cavernous),* may be used interchangeably with fossa. Cavity tends to be more enclosed, fossa a shallower bowl-like space (Orbital fossa-Orbital cavity).
Cavum	A cave.
Cephalic	Pertaining to the head.
Cervico	Pertaining to the Neck.
Clinoid	Like a bed-post, part of a four poster bed so that clinoid processes look like bed posts eg. in the Sphenoid bone.
Clivus	A slope hence in the anterior cranial fossa referring to a slope on the base of the cavity.
Cochlea	A snail, hence snail-like shape relating to the Organ of Corti in the ear.
Compact bone =	**Cortical bone = Dense bone**
	Bone found in the shafts and on external bone surfaces. Highly structured in concentric circles or Haversian systems. It is constantly changing and remodeling depending upon the lines of force.
Concha	A shell shaped bone as in the ear or nose *(pl. conchae adj.-. chonchoid)* old term for this turbinate.
Condyle	A rounded enlargement or process possessing an articulating surface.
Cornu	A horn (as in the Hyoid).
Corona	A crown. *adj.- coronary, coronoid or coronal;* hence a coronal plane is parallel to the main arch of a crown which passes from ear to ear *(c.f. coronal suture).*
Costa / Costo	Pertaining to the ribs.
Cranium	The cranium of the skull comprises all of the bones of the skull except for the mandible.
Crest	Prominent sharp thin ridge of bone formed by the attachment of muscles particularly powerful ones eg Temporalis/Sagittal crest.
Cribiform	A sieve or bone with small sieve-like holes. Ethmoid.
Cuneate/Cuneus	A wedge / wedge-shaped.
Dens	A tooth hence dentine and dental relating to teeth, denticulate having tooth-like projections *adj.- dentate* See also odontoid.
Depression	A concavity on a surface.
Detrition	Wearing away of the tooth surfaces of OA.

Detritus	The material left after the wearing away or rubbing.
Diaphysis	The shaft or body of a long bone. In the young this is the region b/n the growth plates and is composed of compact bone. *pl.- diaphyses adj.- diaphyseal.*
Diploë	The cancellous bone between the inner and outer tables of the skull, *adj.- diploic*.
Edentulous	Without teeth.
Eminence	A smooth projection or elevation on a bone.
Endocranium	Refers to the interior of the "braincase" *adj.- endocranial* divided into the 3 major fossae anterior (for the Frontal lobes) middle (containing Temporal lobes) and posterior (for the containment of the Cerebellum).
Endostium	A mesodermal CT which lines the inner surface of all bones and is the conduit for the NS and BS of the bone llifting of the endostium causes cancellous bone to be laid down to fill the gap b/n the bone and the cellular layer and this device may be used to encourage bone growth/repair. *See periosteum.*
Ethmoid =	**Cribiform.**
External Auditory Meatus	Ear hole.
Exostosis	A bony outgrowth from a bony surface, often due to irritation (as in Swimmer's ear) and may involve ossification of surrounding tissues such as muscles or ligaments.
Facet	A face, a small bony surface (occlusal facet on the chewing surfaces of the teeth) seen in planar joints.
Falciform	Relating to shapes that are in a sickle shape so falciform ligaments curve around and end in a sharp point.
Fissure	A narrow slit or gap from cleft.
Fontanelle	A fountain, associated with the palpable pulsation of the brain as in the anterior fontanelle of an infant. These soft spots on the skull are cartilagenous CT covering "joints" which allow for skull cranial expansion and then become the mould for the bone development and shape joining along the sutural lines, later becoming the Bregma.
Foramen	A natural hole in a bone usually for the transmission of BS and/or nerves. *pl. foramina*.
Fornix	An arch.
Fossa	A pit, depression, or concavity, on a bone, or formed from several bones as in temporomandibular fossa. Shallower and more like a "bowl" than a cavity. *pl. fossae.*
Fovea	A small pit (usually smaller than a fossa)- as in the fovea of the occlusal surface of the molar tooth.
Gallus / Galli	A cock, hence, crista galli, the cock's comb *(i.e. possessive form of gallus)*.
Groove	Long pit or furrow.
Hyoid	U-shaped.
Hyperostosis	Abnormal bone growth generally overgrowth or ectopic growth.
Incisura	A notch.
Inter	Between.
Intra	Within.

Introitus	An orifice or point of entry to a cavity or space.
Joint =	**Articulation + supporting structures.**
Jugum	A bridge between 2 halves of a bone *pl. juga* as in Sphenoid.
Kyphosis	Collapse of vertebral body(ies) causing sharp convexity of the spine.
Lacerum	Something lacerated, mangled or torn e.g. foramen lacerum a small sharp hole at the base of the skull. This often destroys tissues.
Lacrimal	Related to tears and tear drops. *(noun lacrima)*.
Lambda	From the Greek letter a capital 'L' and written as an inverted V. *(adj.- lambdoid)* and used to name the point of connection b/n the 3 skull bones Occipital and Temporals.
Lamellar bone =	**Haversian system.**
	Bone with sheets of concentric collagen fibres around Haversian canals in compact bone.
Lamina	A plate as in the lamina of the vertebra, a plate of bone connecting the vertical and transverse spines *(pl. laminae)*.
Ligament	A band of tissue which connects bones (articular ligaments) or viscera - organs (visceral ligaments). A Ligament is a tie or a connection. Originally *sing. ligamentum pl. ligamenta* from ligate or to tie up is generally composed of collagen fibres. *See classification of ligaments.*
Linea	A line as in the Nuchal lines of the Occipit/Occipital bone.
Lingual	Pertaining to the tongue.
Lipping	Bone projecting over the usual margin, excessive production generally pathological as in osteoarthritis, may interfere with joint movement.
Locus	A place *(c.f. location, locate, dislocate)*.
Lordosis	Increased cervical and/ or lumbar curve also called 'sway back'.
Magnum	Large *pl. magna.*
Malleus	Hammer (as in the ear ossicle).
Mandible	From the verb to chew, hence, the movable lower jaw; *adj.- mandibular.*
Mastoid	A breast or teat shape - mastoid process of the Temporal bone.
Maxilla	The jaw-bone; now used only for the upper jaw; *adj.- maxillary.*
Meatus	A short passage; *adj.- meatal* as in external acoustic meatus connecting the outer ear with the middle ear.
Meniscus	*Gk. crescent.*
Mental	Relating to the chin (mentum = chin, not mens = mind).
Meta	An extension of: cf. metacarpal = extension of the wrist.
Metaphysis =	**Epiphysis** The slightly expanded end of the shaft of a bone. (pl. metaphysis).
Neurocranium	The neurocranium refers only to the braincase of the skull.
Notch	An indentation in the margin of a structure.
Nucha	The nape or back of the neck *adj.- nuchal.*
Occiput	The prominent convexity of the back of the head Occipitum = ccipital bone *adj.- occipital.*
Oculus	An eye *adj.- ocular pl oculi*
Odontoid	Relating to teeth, toothlike. *See Dens.*

Ontogeny	The development of an individual growth pattern.
Orbit	A circle; the name given to the bony socket in which the eyeball rotates; *adj.- orbital.*
Orifice	An opening.
Os	A bone or pertaining to bones *adj.- osseus.*
Ossicle	A small bone as in the ear ossicles: stapes (stirrup), incus (anvil) and malleus (hammer).
Osteitis	Inflammation of the bone.
Osteoblasts	Bone cells capable of dividing and laying down matrix - 'baby' osteocytes
Osteochondroma	Bone & cartilagenous tumour benign often arising in the ephyseal plate or line & protrude at right angles, common & asymptomatic.
Osteoclasts	Multinuclear cells which resorb or phagocytose bone = resorption of bone = Giant cells.
Osteocytes	Bone cells incapable of dividing but maintain the extracelluar matrix of the bone.
Osteogenesis	Formation and growth of bone.

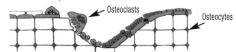

Osteoclasts / Osteocytes

Osteoma	Tumour of the bone tissue.
Osteomalacia	Disease of softening of the bones / Paget's disease. Affects the skull, causing it to enlarge with thick soft bone.
Ostium	A door, an opening, an orifice.
Otic	Pertaining to the ear.
Ovale	Oval shaped.
Palate	A roof *adj.- palatal or platatine.*
Parietal	Pertaining to the outer wall of a cavity from paries, a wall.
Parotid	Pertaining to a region beside or near the ear *(par - otic)*
Pars	A part of / nearby *(adj.- para)*
Pecten	A comb.
Perikymata	Transverse ridges and the grooves on the surfaces of teeth
Periosteum	Layer of fascial tissue (connective tissue) on the outside of compact bone not present on articular (joint) surfaces. *See endostium.*
Periostitis	Inflammation on the outer surface of the bone.
Periostosis	Abnormal growth of long bones on their outer surfaces.
Petrous	Pertaining to a rock / rocky / stoney *adj.- petrosal.*
Phalanx	Pertaining to flanks of soldiers - phalanges a row of soldiers used for a row of fingers or toes.
Planar joints	Joints which allow for sliding across the joint as in the wrist, foot and ribs movement in one plan.
Pneumatic	Air filled *see Classification of Bones.*
Pollex	Thumb.
Process	A general term describing any marked projection or prominence as in the mandibular process.

Prominens	A projection.
Pseudoarthrosis	False or new joint due to the nonhealing of a fracture.
Pterion	A wing; the region where the tip of the greater wing of the sphenoid meets or is close to the parietal, separating the frontal from the squamous region of the temporal bone. (TERY-on) Alternatively the region where these 4 bones meet.
Pterygoid	Wing shaped.
Pubis	Hairy, that part of the hip bone with hair over the surface *adj.- pubic pl. pubes.*
Ramus	Branch as in the superior pubic ramus the superior or higher branch of the pubic bone (Pubis).
Recess	A secluded area or pocket; a small cavity set apart from a main cavity.
Rectus	Straight - erect.
Ridge	Elevated bony growth often roughened.
Rotundum	Round.
Sagittal	An arrow, the sagittal suture is notched posteriorly, making it look like lightning arrows.
Scoliosis	A deviation from the vertical plane of the Vertebral column laterally (as opposed to exaggeration of vertical curves in kyphosis and lordosis).
Sella	A saddle; *adj.- sellar*, sella turcica = Turkish saddle.
Sesamoid	Grainlike.
Sigmoid	S-shaped, from the letter Sigma which is S in Greek.
Sinus	A space usually within a bone, lined with mucous membrane, such as the frontal and maxillary sinuses in the head. A modified BV usually vein, with an enlarged lumen for blood storage & containing no or little muscle in its wall. Sinuses may contain air, venous or arterial blood, lymph or serous fluid depending upon location & health of the subject *adj.- sinusoid*.
Skull	The skull refers to all of the bones that comprise the 'head'.
Spheno-	A wedge i.e. the Sphenoid is the bone which wedges in the base of the skull between the unpaired frontal & occipital bones *adj.- sphenoid*.
Spine	A thorn *adj.- spinous* descriptive of a sharp, slender process/protrusion.
Splanchocranium	The splanchocranium refers to the facial bones of the skull.
Stylos	An instrument for writing hence *adj.- styloid* a pencil-like structure.
Sulcus	Long wide groove often due to a BV indentation.
Sustenaculum	A supportive structure as in the sustenaculum tali = a structure which supports the Talus in the foot.
Suture	The saw-like edge of a cranial bone that serves as joint b/n bones of the skull.
Symphysis	A cartilagenous joint or a growth with bone-cartilage-bone. *See Classification of Joints.*
Syn-	Together i.e... the close proximity of or fusion of 2 structures.
Syndesmosis	Tight inflexible joints b/n 2 bones little to no movement. Many axial joints are of this type.

Synostosis	Fusion of any joints.
Synovial joints	Any moveable joint with synovial fluid b/n the 2 opposing bones - most moving joints are synovial.

Ball & Socket   Condyloid   Hinge

Pivot   Plane   Saddle

Tectum	A roof.
Tegmen	A covering.
Temporal	Refers to time and the fact that grey hair (marking the passage of time) often appears first at the site of the temporal bone.
Tendon	A tie or cord of collagen fibres connecting muscle with bone (as opposed to articular **ligaments** which connect bone with bone).
Tentorium	A tent.
Torus	Protruberance *pl. tori*.
Trabecula	A "little" beam i.e. supporting structure or strut *pl. trabeculae = spicule*.
Trephination	The practice of making an artificial hole in the cranium practiced in many ancient religions used to relieve cranial pressure.
Trochanter	Pertaining to a small wheel or disc. In the femur it is a large disc = shaped tuberosity.
Trochlea	A pulley that part of the bone or ligamentous attachment that pulls the bone in another direction as in the elbow or the ankle (**adj.- Trochlear**).
Tubercle	A small process or bump, an eminence.
Tuberculum	A very small prominence, process or bump.
Tuberosity	A large rounded process or eminence, a swelling or large rough prominence often associated with a tendon or ligament attachment.
Turbinate	A child's spinning top, hence shaped like a top. An old term for the nasal conchae.
Tympanum	A drum *pl. tympani.*
Ulna	= Elbow or arm (*adj.- ulnar*)
Uncus	A hook *adj.- uncinate.*
Wormian bone	Extrasutural bone in the skull.
Zygoma	A yoke, hence the bone joining the maxillary, frontal, temporal & sphenoid bones *adj.- zygomatic*.

*For more medical terms in this or other areas see the **A to Z of Medical terms**.*

Anatomical planes and Anatomical positions

A = Anterior Aspect from the front = or / Posterior Aspect from the back.
Used interchangeably with ventral and dorsal respectively

B = Lateral Aspect from either side

C = Transverse / Horizontal plane

D = Midsagittal plane = Median plane; trunk moving away from this
plane = lateral flexion or lateral movement
plane medial movement;
limbs moving away from this direction = abduction
limbs moving closer to this plane = adduction

E = Coronal plane

F = Median

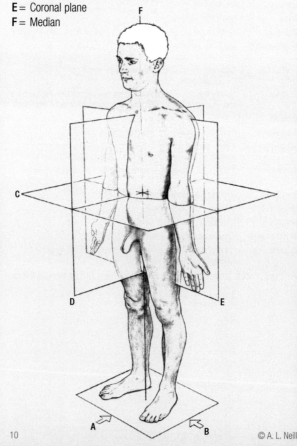

© A. L. Neill

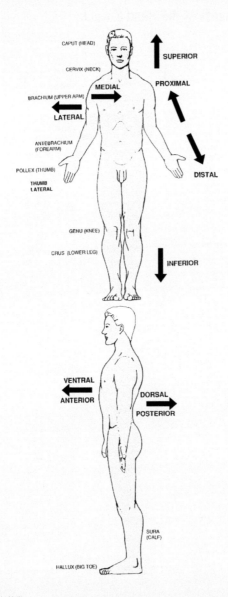

CAPUT (HEAD)

CERVIX (NECK)

SUPERIOR

MEDIAL

PROXIMAL

BRACHIUM (UPPER ARM)

LATERAL

ANTEBRACHIUM
(FOREARM)

DISTAL

POLLEX (THUMB)

**THUMB
LATERAL**

GENU (KNEE)

CRUS (LOWER LEG)

INFERIOR

VENTRAL

ANTERIOR

DORSAL

POSTERIOR

SURA
(CALF)

HALLUX (BIG TOE)

Movements of the Head & Neck

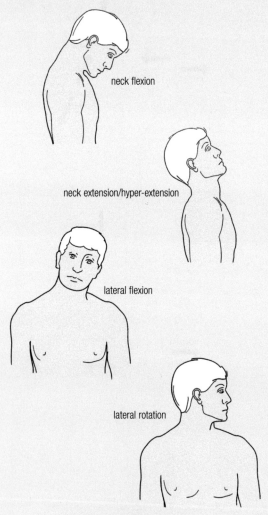

neck flexion

neck extension/hyper-extension

lateral flexion

lateral rotation

note: extension of the neck is in the
normal anatomical position

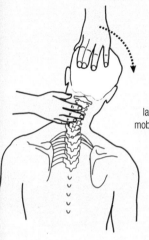

lateral flexion - testing for
mobility and spinal tenderness

cervical flexion - testing for
mobility and spinal tenderness

lateral rotation - testing for
mobility and spinal tenderness

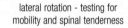

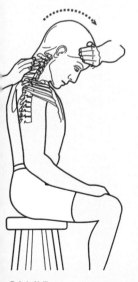

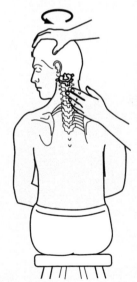

Movements of the Head & Neck Cont/

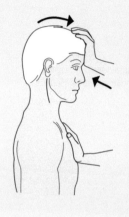

neck flexion - testing for
strength against R

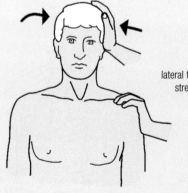

lateral flexion - testing for
strength against R

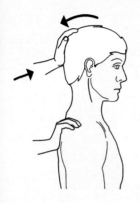

extension / hyperextension - testing for strength against R

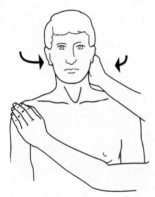

lateral rotation - testing for strength against R

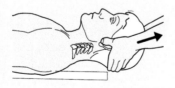

cervical traction - testing for R and N irritation

Movements of the Head & Neck Cont/

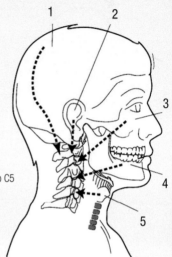

sites of referred pain in
the cervical spine

scalp (1) to SP of C2
ear (2) to body of C2
face (3) to C3
jaw and teeth (4) to C3/4
thyroid, cricoid cartilages (5) to C5

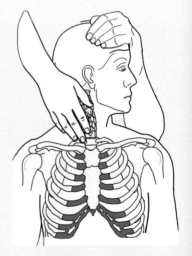

testing for mobility of
C7/T1 and the first rib

© A. L. Neill

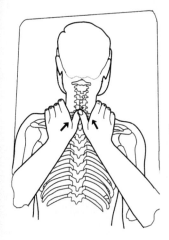

examination for tenderness of
the cervical spinous processes

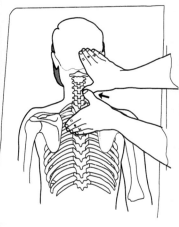

examination for tenderness
of the cervical
transverse processes

The Skull & Neck

Cavities of the Skull

Cervical Spine Radiological Overview

Articulations of the Skull bones

Bones	Paired	ear	eth	fro	hy	lac	mn	max	nas	occ	pal	par	sphn	temp	vom	zyg	C1 C2
ear ossicles = ear	Yes																
ethmoid = eth	No			•		•		•	•		•		•		•		
frontal = fro	No		•			•		•	•			•	•			•	
hyoid = hy	No																
lacrimal = lac	Yes		•	•				•									
mandible = mn	No													•			
maxilla = max	Yes		•	•		•			•		•				•	•	
nasal = nas	Yes		•	•				•									
occipital = occ	No											•	•	•			•
palatine = pal	Yes		•					•					•		•		
parietal = par	Yes			•						•			•	•			
sphenoid = sphn	No		•	•						•	•	•		•	•	•	
temporal = temp	Yes						•			•		•	•			•	
vomer = vom	No		•					•			•		•				
zygoma = zyg	Yes			•				•					•	•			

Red spots indicate when there is an articulation or joint between the bones. Please note the hyoid does not articulate with any bones and the mandible articulates at the only synovial joint in the skull- the TMJ -temporomandibular joint. All other joints are secondary cartilagenous bone-fibrocartilage-bone.

Skull Bones External Views
Face

Bones as they affect the face - surface projection

anterior

1 Frontal bone

2 Superciliary arch

3 Supra-orbital notch

4 Glabella

5 Nasion – fronto-nasal suture

6 Maxilla

7 Nasal bone

8 Zygoma

9 Fronto-zygomatic suture

10 Cheek prominence

11 Zygomatic arch

12 Infraorbital foramen

13 Angle of the jaw

14 Mental foramen

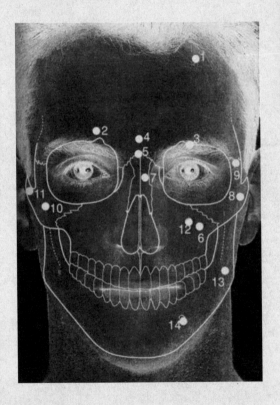

Skull External Views

anterior

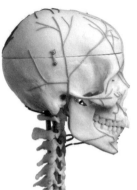

1   Frontal bone
2   Fronto-nasal suture
3   Inter-nasal suture
4   Nasal bone
5   Supra-orbital foramen
6   Spheno-parietal suture
7   Spheno-frontal suture
8   Spheno-squamosal suture
9   Zygoma
10 Zygomatico-maxillary suture
11 Infra-orbital foramen
12 Middle nasal concha – turbinate
13 Inferior nasal concha – turbinate
14 Vomer
15 Mandible
16 Mental foramen
17 Inter-maxillary suture
18 Maxilla
19 Ethmoid bone (orbital plate)
20 Inferior orbital fissure
21 Temporo-zygomatic suture
22 Superior orbital fissure
23 Fronto-zygomatic suture
24 Greater wing of the sphenoid
25 Coronal suture - Fronto-parietal suture
26 Lesser wing of the sphenoid
27 Optic foramen

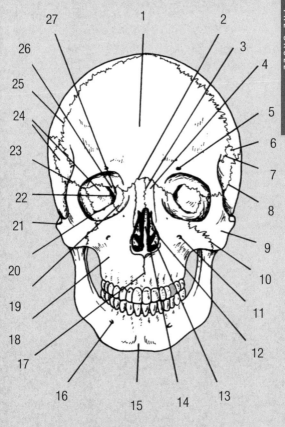

27

26

25

24

23

22

21

20

19

18

17

16

1

2

3

4

5

6

7

8

9

10

11

12

13

14

15

External Skull

Anterior

radiology occipitofrontal

1 Sagittal suture

2 Lambdoid suture (view to the posterior) meeting at the Bregma

3 Frontal sinus

4 Lesser wing of the sphenoid

5 Supra-orbital fissure

6 Greater wing of the sphenoid

7 Fronto-zygomatic suture

8 Petrous ridge

9 Anterior clinoid process

10 Floor of the hypophyseal fossa + upper apex of nasal cavity adjacent to nasal sinuses

11 Lateral pterygoid plate

12 Base of the skull - floor of posterior cranial cavity

13 Foramen rotundum

14 Mastoid process

15 Upper central incisor tooth

16 Mandible

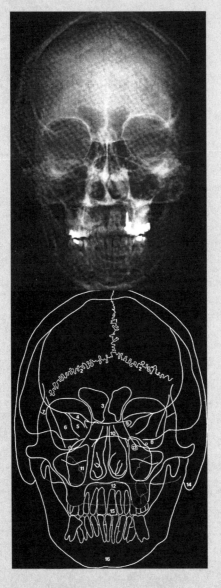

External Skull

Anterior

upper and lower views in detail
radiology occipitofrontal (upper)

1 Frontal sinus

2 Ethmoid sinus

3 Maxillary sinus

4 Foramen rotundum

5 Supra-orbital fissure

6 Anterior clinoid process

7 Posterior clinoid process

8 Petrous ridge

9 Floor of the hypophyseal fossa + upper apex of nasal cavity adjacent to nasal sinuses

10 Crista galli

11 Frontal process of zygoma

12 Middle concha - turbinate

13 Inferior concha - turbinate

14 Lateral border of Greater wing of the sphenoid

15 Greater wing of the sphenoid

16 Lesser wing of the sphenoid

17 Hard palate

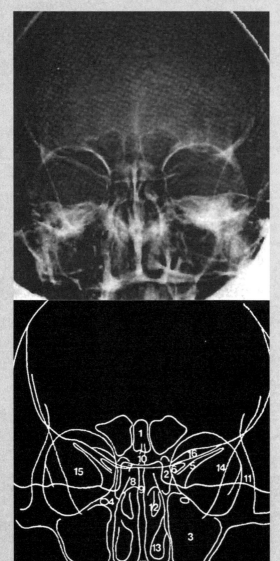

External Skull

Anterior

upper and lower views in detail
radiology occipitomental (lower)

1 Frontal sinus

2 Ethmoid sinus

3 Maxillary sinus

4 Foramen rotundum

5 Supra-orbital fissure

6 Anterior clinoid process

7 Posterior clinoid process

8 Petrous ridge

9 Floor of the hypophyseal fossa + upper apex of nasal cavity adjacent to nasal sinuses

10 Crista galli

11 Frontal process of zygoma

12 Middle concha - turbinate

13 Inferior concha - turbinate

14 Lateral border of Greater wing of the sphenoid

15 Greater wing of the sphenoid

16 Lesser wing of the sphenoid

17 Hard palate

18 Infra-orbital foramen

19 Zygomatico-facial foramen

20 Coronoid process of the mandible

21 Soft tissue of lower lid

22 Pterygoid plates of the sphenoid

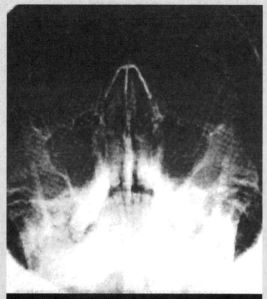

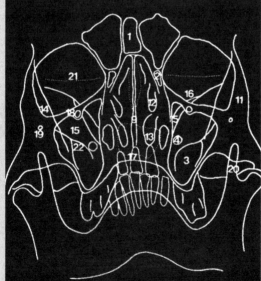

Skull External Views

inferior base of skull

1 Incisive fossa - alveolare
2 Medial pterygoid plate and Hamulus
3 Posterior nasal aperture
4 Maxillary process of Zygoma
5 Lateral Pterygoid plate
6 Zygomatic arch
7 Mandibular fossa
8 External Auditory Meatus
9 Styloid process
10 Mastoid process
11 Parieto-mastoid suture
12 Occipito-mastoid suture
13 Foramen magnum
14 External occipital protruberance
15 Sagittal suture - Parieto-parieto suture
16 Lambda
17 Lambda suture
18 Superior nuchal line (Occipital)
19 Inferior nuchal line (Occipital)
20 Occipital condyle
21 Jugular foramen (fossa)
22 Stylo-mastoid foramen
23 Carotid foramen - carotid canal
24 Foramen spinosum
25 Foramen lacerum - basilar suture
26 Greater palatine foramen
27 Horizontal plate of palatine
28 Palatine process of the maxilla

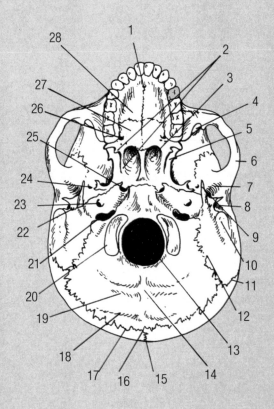

28
27
26
25
24
23
22
21
20
19
18
17 16 15
1
2
3
4
5
6
7
8
9
10
11
12
13
14

External Skull

Inferior

radiology submentovertical view

1 Nasal septum
2 Posterior border of vomer
3 Maxillary sinus
4 Ethmoid sinus
5 Greater palatine foramen
6 Lesser palatine foramen
7 Sphenoid sinus
8 Posterior orbital margin - greater wing of the sphenoid
9 Posterior boundary of the maxillary sinus
10 Zygomatic arch
11 Lesser wing of the sphenoid
12 Head of mandible condyloid process
13 Foramen ovalae
14 Foramen spinosum
15 Spine of the sphenoid
16 Foramen lacerum
17 Clivus - base of the occipital & sphenoid bones
18 Eustachian tube - (auditory tube)
19 Carotid canal
20 Jugular foramen
21 Stylomastoid foramen
22 Anterior arch of the atlas (C1)
23 Odontoid process of axis (C2)
24 Occipital condyles
25 Foramen magnum
26 Canaliculus for tympanic N
27 Inner and outer tables of the skull - Diploe

THE SKULL

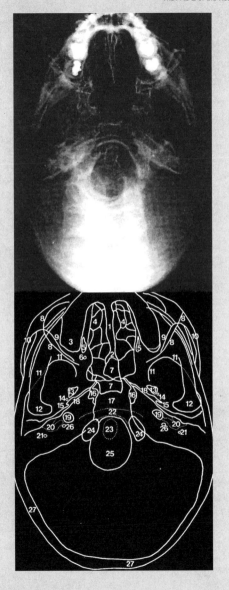

Skull External Views

Infero-lateral / Oblique

1 Zygoma a = arch of

2 Orbital fossa

3 Nasal bone

4 Incisive fossa = Alveolare

5 Hard palate

6 Pterygoid plate L = lateral m = medial

7 Scaphoid fossa

8 Styloid process

9 Mastoid process

10 Temporal bone p= petrous part of

11 Foramen magnum

12 Occiptum c= condyle of

13 Eustachian tube = auditory tube

14 EAM

15 Sphenoid bone

16 Frontal bone

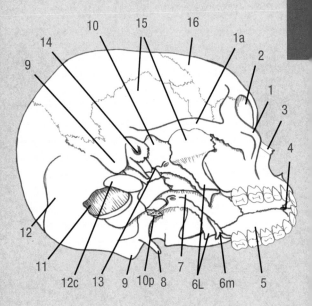

Skull External Views

lateral

1 Frontal bone - temporal ridges for attachment of Temporalis (aka temporal lines)

2 Parietal bone

3 Occipital bone

4 Mastoid process

5 Temporal bone

6 Zygomatic arch

7 Mandible

8 Body of mandible

9 Maxilla

10 Zygoma

11 Nasal bone

12 Lacrimal bone

13 Frontal bone

14 Greater wing of the sphenoid

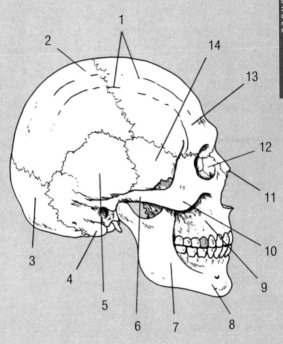

External Skull

Lateral / oblique

radiology

1 Coronal suture

2 Impression for middle meningeal artery

3 Lambdoid suture

4 Wormian bone - extrasutural bone

5 Styloid process

6 Posterior wall of nasopharynx

7 Clivus - (base of sphenoid and occipital bones)

8 Hypophyseal fossa

9 Sphenoid sinus

10 Greater wing of the sphenoid

11 Posterior air cells in the ethmoid - ethmoid sinus

12 Anterior air cells in the ethmoid - ethmoid sinus

13 Frontal sinus

14 Zygoma - frontal process

15 Maxilla - malar process

16 Zygoma - arch

17 Posterior border of the maxillary sinus

18 Hard palate - palatine bone

19 Alveolar bone in maxilla

20 Pterygoid plates

21 Soft tissue of soft palate and uvula

22 Mandibular canal

23 Head of mandible

24 Coronoid process of mandible

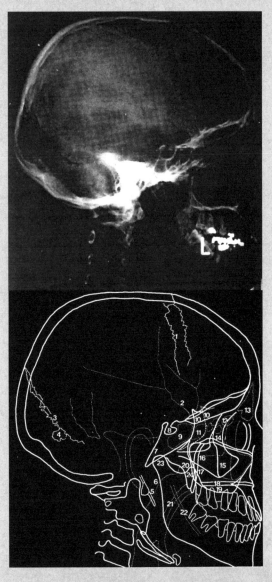

Skull External Views

Postero-inferior – rear view with tilt
Mandible attached – rear view of the TMJ

1 Sutural bones = Inca = Wormian bones enclosed in the skull sutures

2 Parietal bones

3 Nuchal lines i = inferior s = superior

4 Foramen magnum

5 Mastoid process

6 Sphenoid bone s = spine of

7 Pterygoid plate L = lateral m = medial

8 Incisive fossa = alveolare= ant. palatine fossa

9 Digastric fossa = attachment for geniohyoid

10 Mental spines inf. & superior (muscle attachments)

11 Mandible

12 Hard palate

13 Greater palatine foramen

14 Hypoglossal canal

15 Nasal turbinates = conchae sup., middle & inf.

16 Styloid process (temporal bone)

17 Zygomatic arch

18 Temporal bone

19 Occipitum

see also the Nasal Cavity & TMJ

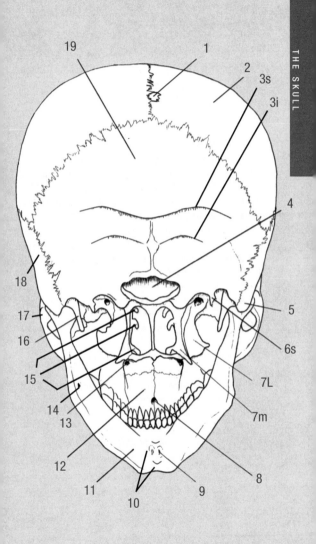

Skull External Views

Posterior
Superior (skull cap)

1 Sagittal suture (over the sagittal sinus – venous blood in the skull)

2 Parietal bone
   E = parietal eminence = Euryon
   f = foramen

3 Lambda = meeting point of parietal bones & occiput

4 Lambdoid suture (parieto-occipital suture)

5 Occiput / p = external occipital protruberance

6 Temporal bone with mastoid process

7 7i =Inferior nuchal line 7s= superior nuchal line

8 Incisive fossa = Alveolare of the hard palate

9 Hard palate

10 Sutural bones = Wormian bones = Inca

11 Frontal bone

12 Coronal suture (parieto-frontal suture)

13 Bregma (∩ Coronal & Sagittal sutures)

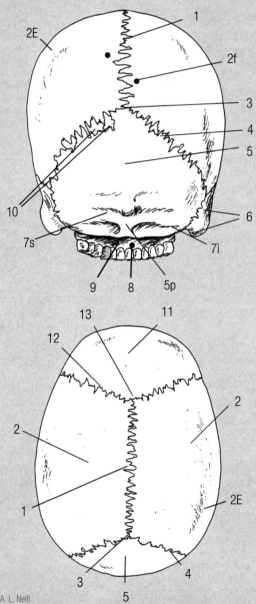

Skull Internal Views

Inferior Skull cap

1 Lambda

2 Lambdoid suture

3 Parietal foramen

4 Diploe

5 Bregma

6 Coronal suture

7 Frontal crest

8 Frontal bone

9 Depressions for arachnoid granulations

10 Grooves for middle meningeal vessels

11 Parietal bone

12 Sagittal suture

13 Groove for superior sagittal sinus

14 Occipital bone

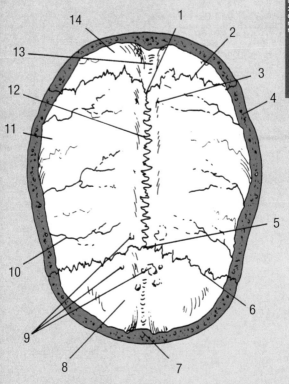

Skull Internal Views

Lateral - looking out to the sides of the skull from the inside

1 Groove for the middle meningeal artery

2 Frontal sinus

3 Superior nasal concha

4 Middle nasal concha

5 Inferior nasal concha

6 Hard palate

7 Mandible

8 Lateral pterygoid plate

9 Medial pterygoid plate

10 Styloid process

11 Mastoid process

12 Sphenoid sinus

For medial view of the Nasal area - nasal septum see Nasal bones and cavity

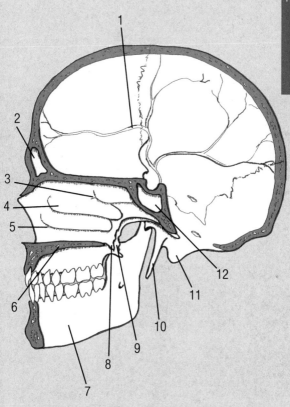

Skull Internal Views
Superior internal base - cranial fossae

1 Cribiform plate
2 Frontal sinus
3 Crista Galli
4 Orbital plate of frontal bone
5 Jugum of sphenoid
6 Optic canal
7 Lesser wing of the sphenoid bone
8 Anterior clinoid process
9 Foramen rotundum
10 Foramen lacerum
11 Foramen ovale
12 Foramen spinosum
13 Dorsum sellae
14 Internal acoustic meatus
15 Jugular foramen
16 Foramen magnum

A ANTERIOR FOSSA
B MIDDLE FOSSA
C POSTERIOR FOSSA

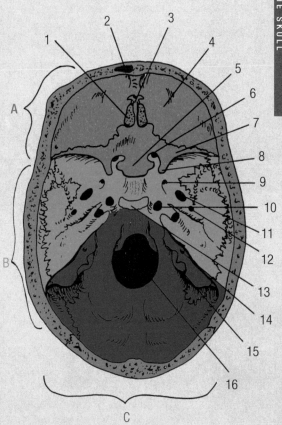

Maxillary Sinus (Left)

Sagittal

1 Frontal sinus

2 Anterior ethmoidal foramen

3 Orbital plate of the ethmoid

4 Posterior ethmoidal foramen

5 Lesser wing of the sphenoid

6 Pterygo-maxillary fissure

7 Perpendicular plate of the palatine

8 Alveolar processes of the maxilla

9 Maxillary sinus - opened

10 Inferior concha

11 Anterior nasal spine

12 Uncinate process of the ethmoid

13 Nasal bone

14 Lacrimo-maxillary suture

15 Supra-orbital foramen

16 Frontal bone

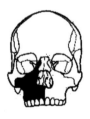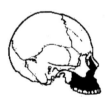

Description: Maxilla - sinuses within this bone - particularly around the teeth may cause toothache, complicate endodontic (root canal) treatment; or act as a conduit for tooth/nasal/other infection to enter the blood stream.

CAVITIES OF THE SKULL

© A. L. Neill

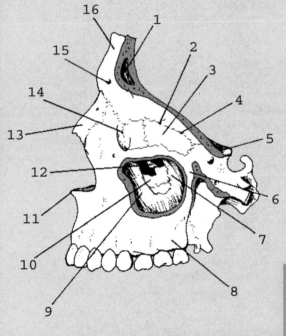

16

15

14

13

1

2

3

4

5

6

7

8

9

10

11

12

Orbital Cavity / Fossa (Left)

Anterior view

1 Lesser wing of the sphenoid

2 Optic foramen

3 Anterior and posterior ethmoidal foramina

4 Lacrimal bone

5 Nasal bone

6 Orbital plate of the ethmoid bone

7 Orbital plate of the maxilla

8 Infra-orbital foramen

9 Infra-orbital groove

10 Zygoma

11 Inferior orbital fissure

12 Foramina for zygomatic branch of the facial nerve

13 Orbital surface of the zygoma

14 Greater wing of the sphenoid

15 Superior orbital fissure

16 Orbital plate of the frontal bone

17 Supra-orbital margin

18 Supra-orbital foramen

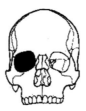

Eyeball and muscles all sit in this cavity with the Optic nerve entering from the posterior part of the cavity through the Orbital foramen.

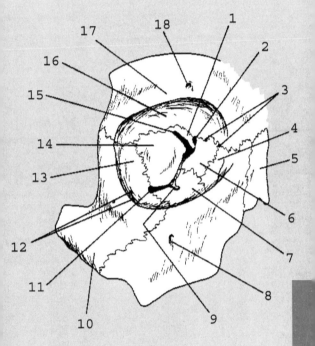

Orbital cavity

Inferoanterior

radiology (also Orbital fossa / Optic cavity / Optic foramen)

1 Frontal sinus

2 Foramen ovale

3 Infra-orbital foramen

4 Foramen rotundum

5 Hard palate – floor of nasal cavity

6 Maxillary antrum

7 Lateral wall of maxillary antrum

8 Zygomatic arch

9 Sphenoid sinus

10 Soft tissue of nose and lower lid

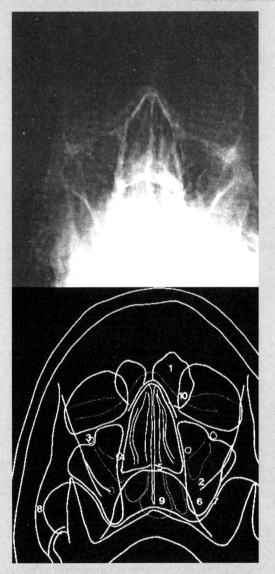

Paranasal sinuses = Sinuses

Coronal

The paranasal sinuses are generally the "sinuses" referred to when discussing sinus pain etc - they are the air filled spaces which empty into the nasal cavity. They may swell, become infected and fill with fluid, causing pain and pathology. A number of bones contribute to this space, as indicated.

1 Cranial vault (ACF at this point)

2 Ethmoid air cells

3 Maxillary sinus

4 Nasal cavity

5 Boney palate = hard palate

6 Inferior meatus (opening)
6A Inferior concha (turbinate)

7 Middle meatus
7A Middle concha (turbinate)

8 Superior meatus
8A Superior concha (turbinate)

9 Orbit / orbital fossa

■ Contribution of the frontal bone

■ Contribution of the zygoma

■ **Contribution of the maxilla**

■ Contribution of the ethmoid bone

■ Inferior nasal concha (is its own bone)

■ **Vomer**

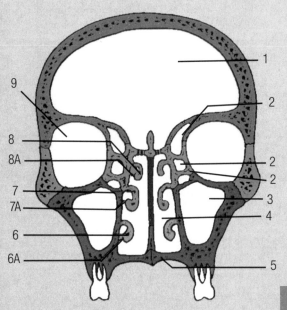

Paranasal sinuses = Sinuses

Coronal – Frontal
Transverse

Radiology

The paranasal sinuses are generally the "sinuses" referred to when discussing sinus pain etc - they are the air filled spaces which empty into the nasal cavity and communicate with each other with many variations.

They may become involved in the spread of infection and cancer throughout the Head, Face and Cranial cavities.

1 Cranial vault (ACF at this point)

2 Frontal sinus

3 Ethmoid sinuses / spaces
a = ant. cells / p = post. cells
i = infundibulum leading to the maxillary sinus (5)
pp = perpendicular plate
u = uncinate process

4 floor of the orbital cavity –
c = infra-orbital canal
s = additional sinus in the floor of the orbit – varies

5 Maxillary sinus

6 Nasal conchae
i = inf. nasal concha
m = middle nasal concha
s = superior nasal concha

7 Vomer

8 Nasal septum
t = tubercle i.e. some septi have swellings & overgrowths as well as deviations interfering with breathing

9 Middle nasal meatus (opening)

10 Orbital cavity showing eyeball and peri-orbital fat

11 Crista galli – this one pneumatised (air filled) – varies

12 Lateral rectus

13 Sphenoid sinuses

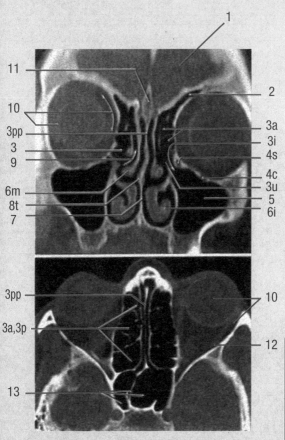

1

11

10

3pp

3

9

6m

8t

7

2

3a

3i

4s

4c

3u

5

6i

3pp

3a,3p

13

10

12

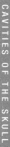

Neck

Anterior-Posterior

radiology

1 Body of C3

2 Transverse processes - C5, C6, C7

3 First rib

4 Transverse process - T1

5 Spinous processes - C4, C5, C6

Neck

Open Mouth - Dens process

radiology

1 Occipital condyles

2 Lateral mass of C1

3 Dens process (C2)

4 Body of C2

5 Spinous processes C2, C3

6 Occiput

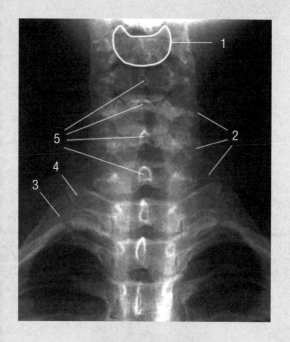

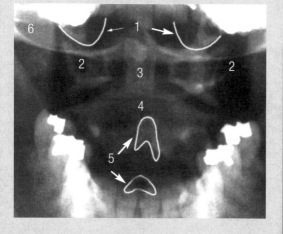

Neck

Anterior-Oblique

radiology

1 Dens

2 Body of C2

3 Body of C3

4 Body of C4

5 Body of C5

6 Body of C6

7 Body of C7

8 First rib

9 Inferior articulating processes

10 Intervertebral foraminae C2/3, C3/4

11 Pedicles

12 Superior articulating processes

13 Spinous processes C5, C6

14 Second rib

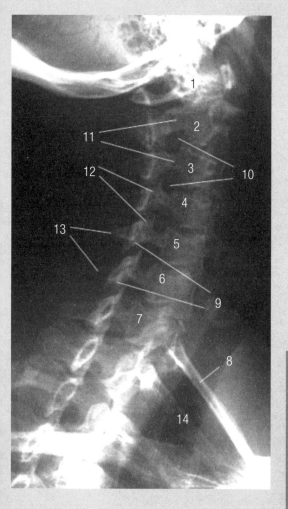

Neck

Lateral

radiology

1   Occipital condyles

2   Anterior arch of C1

3   Dens process (C2)

4   Body of C2

5   Zygapophyseal joints = facet joints

6   Intervertebral space - intervertebral discs (radiologically lucent)

7   Inferior articulating surfaces

8   Vertebral bodies C6, C7, T1

9   Pedicles

10 Spinous processes

11 Lamina

12 Superior articulating processes

13 Posterior arch of C1

14 Occiput

CAVITIES OF THE SKULL

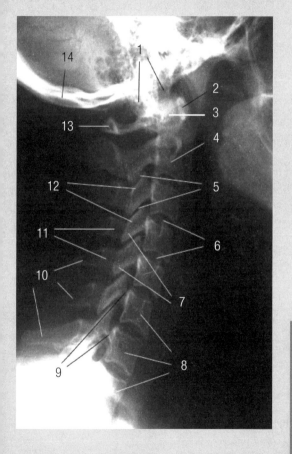

Bones, Cartilages, Joints & Ligaments, Overviews

© A. L. Neill

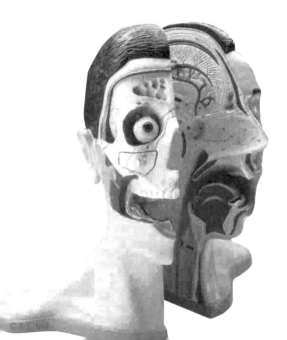

©A. L. Neill

CAVITIES OF THE SKULL

A Atlas = C1 = First Cervical Vertebra

B *anterior / superior*

C *(Atlas - Gk demigod who held up the world on his shoulders).*

Articulations:	Atlanto-Axial jts (3)	C1-C2
	Atlanto-Occipital jts (2)	C1-Occiput (Base of the skull)
Special features	no vertebral body no spinous process no articular discs	special anterior facet for dens (odontoid process)

1 Facet for odontoid / dens process

2 Ant. tubercle

3 Superior articular facet

4 Inferior articular facet

5 Posterior tubercle

6 Posterior arch

7 Groove for vertebral BVs & suboccipital N

8 Foramen transversarium = transverse foramen

9 TP

10 Lat. mass

11 Vertebral foramen

12 Ant. arch

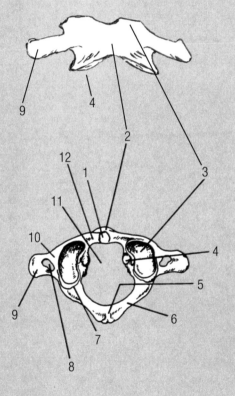

A **Atlanto - Axial joint -** *median =*

ODONTOID JOINT *aka hanging joint*

BS spinal branches of vertebral art.

NS spinal Ns dorsal rami (C1-2)

A rotation, circumduction

Atlanto-Axial joints - *lateral =*

zygapophyseal joints of C1/C2

BS spinal branches of vertebral art.

NS spinal Ns dorsal rami (C1-2)

A flexion, extension, lateral flexion, rotation

1 Dens = odontoid process (C2)

2 Transverse lig of axis (C2)

3 Transverse foramen of atlas C1

4 Medial tubercle of atlas (C1)

5 Tranverse foramen of axis (C2)

6 Post arch and tubercle of atlas (C1)

7 Lamina and spine of axis (C2)

8 Body of axis (C2)

9 Superior articular facet of atlanto-occipital jt

10 Ant. arch of atlas (C1)

11 Facet for dens (C2)

12 Ant. tubercle of atlas (C1)

Atlanto-Occipital joint (see Craniovertebral joint)

A B C D E F G H I J K L M N O P Q R S T U V W X Y Z

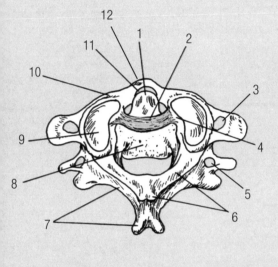

A Auditory ossicles = Ear bones - middle ear (in the Temporal bone)

Overview - In situ - individual bones

Description - 3 bones incus = anvil, malleus = hammer, stapes = stirrup in the temporal bone middle ear cavity. Malleus abuts the tympanic membrane of the middle ear (eardrum) articulates with the incus and then the stapes which abuts to the round window

Articulations:	Malleo-Incus	Hammer with the eardrum
	Incus-Stapes	inter ear ossicle articulation
	Stapo - Temporal	stirrup with the temporal bone round membrane
Special features	small bones with delicate balance to transmit sound	articulate with membrane stretched across bone at both ends

1 External Auditory Meatus = earhole

2 External ear

3 Tympanic membrane = lateral border for the middle ear

4 Inner ear

5 Auditory tube

6 Cochlea

7 Cochlea N

8 Facial N

9 Vestibular N

10 Oval window with stapes

11 Vestibular canals

12 Incus

13 Malleus

14 Promontory

15 Round window

View of individual bones actual size. Right and Left sides respectively from above down Stapes Incus Malleus

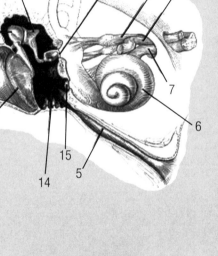

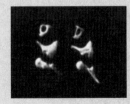

A Axis = C2 = Second Cervical Vertebra

anterior / superior

(Axis - pivot for movement of the head, all movements but nodding)

Articulations:	Atlanto-Axial jts (3)	C1-C2
	vertebro-axial Axial jts (2) (Base of the skull)	C1-Occiput
Special features	no vertebral body dens/odontoid process no articular discs	Dens acts as an AXIS for rotation at C1

1 Dens = odontoid process (tooth)
2 Attachment of alar ligament
3 Groove for transverse ligament
4 Pedicle
5 Body
6 Vertebral foramen
7 Spinous process
8 Lamina
9 Inferior articular process
10 Transverse process
11 Transverse notch / foramen (if closed)
12 Superior articular facet
13 Facet for odontoid / dens process

CHEEK BONES (see Zygoma)
CHIN (see Mandible)

A
B
C
D
E
F
G
H
I
J
K
L
M
N
O
P
Q
R
S
T
U
V
W
X
Y
Z

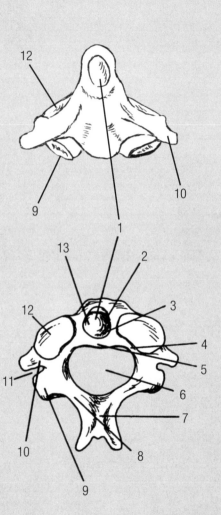

A # Craniovertebral joints = HEAD/SPINE joints

B *anterior*

C *(made up of median and lateral Atlanto-Occipital (C1/head) and Axial-*
D *Occipital joints (C2/head) joints)*

E **BS** *vertebral arteries*

F **NS** *medial branches of dorsal rami, recurrent laryngeal*
spinal branches of ventral rami (C1-3)
G

H **A** *flexion/extension, lateral flexion, rotation*

I 1 Basilar of occiput

J 2 Jugular foramen (transverse foramen in the base of
K the skull)

L 3 Mastoid process

M 4 Transverse process of C1

N 5 ALL = anterior longitudinal lig, attached to tubercle
O of atlas

P 6 Intervertebral disc C2, C3

Q 7 ALL
R

S 8 C2/C3 zygapophyseal joint

T 9 Capsule of the lateral atlanto-occipital joint

U 10 Capsule of the lateral atlanto-axial joint

V 11 Ant. atlanto-occipital membrane

W

X

Y

Z

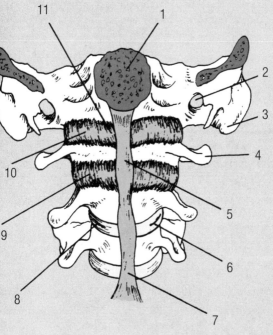

A **Craniovertebral joints = HEAD/SPINE joints**

B *lateral*

C *(made up of median and lateral Atlanto-Occipital (C1/head) and Axial-Occipital joints (C2/head) joints)*

D

E **BS** *vertebral arteries*

F **NS** *medial branches of dorsal rami, recurrent laryngeal spinal branches of ventral rami (C1-3)*

G **A** *flexion/extension, lateral flexion, rotation*

H 1 Basilar of Occiput

I 2 Tectorial membrane

J 3 Ant. atlanto-occipital membrane leads to the (3A)

K 3A ALL

L 4 Apical lig of dens

M 5 Ant. arch of atlas C1

N 6 Dens of C2

7 Longitudinal band of cruciform lig superior (becomes 7A)

O 7A Longitudinal band of cruciform lig inferior

P 8 C2/C3 intervertebral disc

Q 9 Body of C3

R 10 Post. longitudinal lig =PLL

S 11 Lamina of C2

T 12 Transverse lig of atlas (C1)

U 13 Post atlanto-axial lig

V 14 Post arch of C1

15 Vertebral artery

W 16 Post. atlanto-occipital lig

X 17 Space which leads to foramen magnum & then...

Y 17A Vertebral foramen

Z

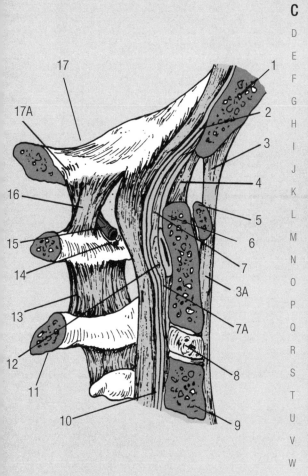

A **Craniovertebral joints = HEAD/SPINE joints**

B *posterior*

C *(made up of median and lateral Atlanto-Occipital (C1/head) and Axial-Occipital joints (C2/head) joints).*

D

BS *vertebral arteries*

E

NS *medial branches of dorsal rami, recurrent laryngeal spinal branches of ventral rami (C1-3)*

F

G **A** *flexion/extension, lateral flexion, rotation*

H 1 Jugular foramen

I 2 Transverse process of atlas

3 Tectoral membrane

J

3A PLL

K

4 Capsule of zygapophyseal joints

L 5 C2/C3 intervertebral disc

M 6 Longitudinal band of cruciform lig inferior

N 7 Capsule of lat. joint of C1 - C2

8 Transverse band of cruciform lig over the deeper stronger transverse lig of the atlas (C1)

O

P

9 Alar lig*

Q

10 Capsule of lat. atlanto-occipital jt

R 11 Longitudinal band of cruciform lig superior

S *broken in hanging*

T

U

V

W

X

Y

Z

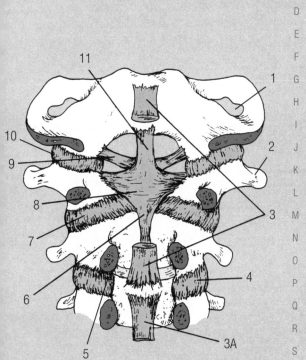

A **EAR BONES = Auditory Ossicles**

B *in situ*

C *middle ear / INCUS, MALLEUS & STAPES*

D
E
F
G
H
I
J
K
L
M
N

1 Head of malleus
2 Body of incus
3 Short process of incus
4 Ant. malleolar process
5 Post. crus of stapes
6 Base of stapes
7 Ant. crus of stapes
8 Long. process of stapes
9 Lenticular process of incus
10 Handle of malleus
11 Ant. process of malleus
12 Neck of malleus
13 Lateral malleolar process

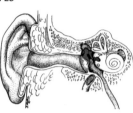

inner ear / cochlea / labyrinth

O
P
Q
R
S
T
U
V
W
X
Y

21 Ant. semicircular canal
22 Ant. bony ampulla
23 Elliptical recess
24 Spherical recess
25 Cochlea
26 Cupola of cochlea
27 Base of cochlea
28 Oval window - fenestra vestibuli
29 Post. bony ampulla
30 Round window - fenestra cochlea
31 Lat. semicircular canal
32 Post. semicircular canal
33 Lat. bony ampulla

Z

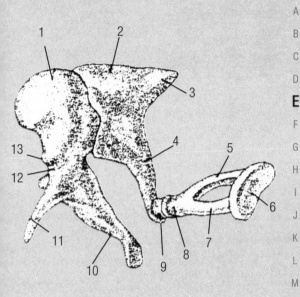

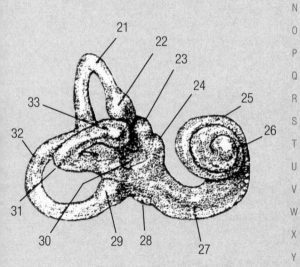

A # Ethmoid bones

B *anterior / lateral / superior / medial*

C *(Ethmoid = sieve, light spongy cubic shaped bone sitting b/n the two
orbital cavities). Part of the paranasal sinuses.*

D

E 1 Ethmoidal labyrinth containing air cells (part of the
ethmoid sinus) continuous with the sphenoid sinus

F

2 Crista galli

G

3 Orbital plate of ethmoid bone (part of the orbital cavity)

H

I 4 Middle nasal concha

J 5 Jugum of sphenoid - jugum sphenoidale (bridge
connecting the two wings of the sphenoid bone)

K

L 6 Perpendicular plate of the palatine bone

M 7 Uncinate process

N

8 Ala (of crista galli)

O

P 9 Anterior groove (on the ethmoid)

Q 10 Posterior groove (on the ethmoid)

R 11 Cribiform plate (entrance for the olfactory nerve)

S 12 Vomer

T

U

V

W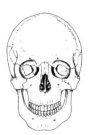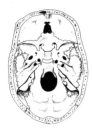

X

Y

Z

© A. L. Neill

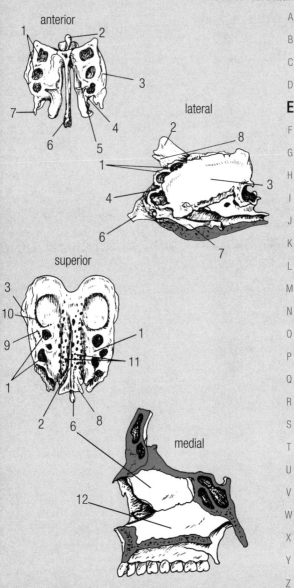

anterior

1
2
3
7
4
6
5

lateral

2
8
1
3
4
6
7

superior

3
10
9
1
1
2
6
8
11

medial

6
12

Frontal bones

anterior / lateral / inferior

Description: Unpaired largest and very robust anterior bone forming the forehead - horizontal section forming the roof of the orbit and contributing to the paranasal sinuses.

1 Frontal tuberosity - frontal bossing

2 Superciliary arch

3 Supra-orbital margin and notch

4 Nasal spine

5 Superior and inferior temporal lines

6 Superior orbital plate - pars orbitalis

7 Frontal and ethmoid air cells

8 Post. ethmoidal foramen

9 Ant. ethmoidal foramen

10 Zygomatic process

11 Supra-orbital notch

12 Lacrimal fossa

13 Metopic suture - frontal suture, glabella

14 Frontal squama

15 Ethmoidal notch

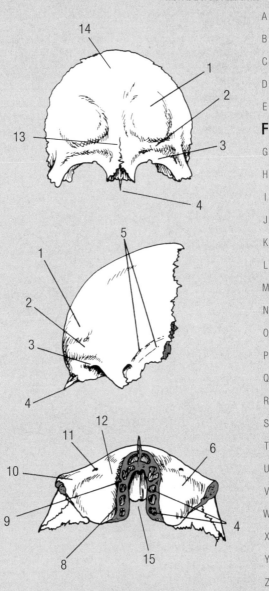

E

Hyoid

B *Description - Small U-shaped bone. Attached to the styloid processes*
via ligaments. This bone has no articulations - the only bone in the
C *body - and is not normally broken in trauma, protected by the*
mandible / CHIN. It may be broken in hanging and strangulation.
D

Articulations:	nil
Special features	of interest in Forensic Ix, rarely broken unless specific pressure on this bone because of its site, acts to shape the jawline by supporting and bending the strap muscles

H

I 1   Body of hyoid

J 2   Greater horn (cornu)

K 3   Lesser horn (cornu)

L
MUSCLE ATTACHMENTS
M

N 4   Genioglossus

5   Geniohyoid
O

P 6   Middle phayngeal constrictor

Q 7   Hypoglossus

R
8   Stylohyoid
S

T 9   Thyrohyoid

U 10 Omohyoid

V 11 Sternohyoid

W 12 Mylohyoid

X
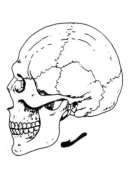
Incus – see Auditory Ossicles
Y

Z

© A. L. Neill

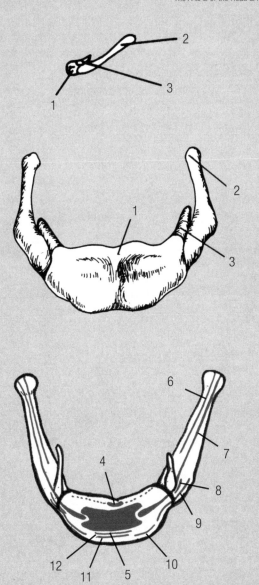

A Inferior Nasal Concha = Inferior Nasal Turbinate

B *Lateral*

Description – small long thin areolar bone covered in mucosal epithelium

Articulations:	with maxilla laterally with ethmoid posteriorly & laterally with lacrimal superiorly	All 2° fibrocartilagenous joints
Special Features	the only nasal concha bone which is an independent	other conchae are formations of the Maxilla

1 Lacrimal process
2 Ethmoidal process
3 Maxillary process

L Lacrimal

M *Description - Small cone-shaped bone.*

Articulations:	with ethmoid laterally with frontal superiorly with inferior nasal concha inferiorly with maxilla medially	All 2° fibrocartilagenous joints

1 Apex – articulates with frontal
2 Lacrimal crest and groove
3 Hammulus
4 Descending process
5 Inferior edge
6 Medial edge

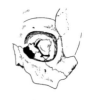

JAW – see Mandible

Malleus – see Auditory Ossicles

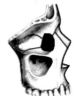

© A. L. Neill

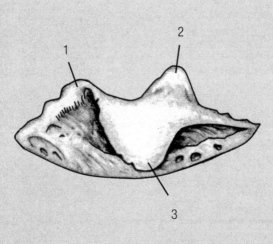

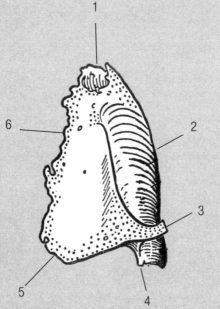

A **Larynx**

B *Cartilages articulated and disarticulated.*

C 1 Hyoid bone

D 2 Epiglottis

E

F 3 Thyroid membrane

G 4 Thyroid cartilage

H 4 Thyroid cartilage
   A = superior horn
I   B = inferior horn

J

K 5 Medial cricothyroid ligament

L 6 Cricoid cartilage

M 7 Arytenoid cartilages

N 8 Tracheal "rings"

O 9 Corniculate cartilages

P

Q 10 Attachment for transverse arytenoid

R 11 Muscular process (for arytneoids)

S 12 Attachment for vocal cords

T

U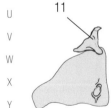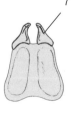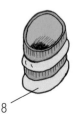

© A. L. Neill

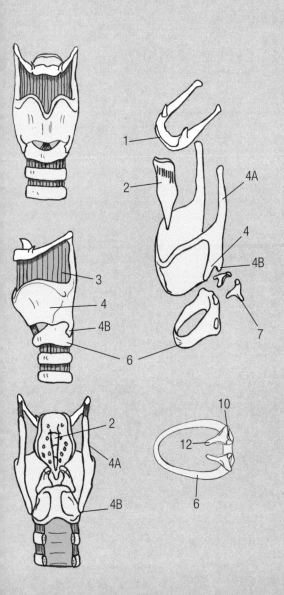

A # Mandible = JAW

B *lateral / posterior*

C *(Mandible - lower jaw bone joins the skull via the condyles and a cartilaginous articular plate in the temporal fossa.*

D *Primary function - mastication, houses all the bottom teeth).*

E
Articulations:	with the temporal fossa - this shallow fossa makes it easy to dislocate this joint	TMJ = temporomandibular joint

H
1   Mandibular notch

I
2   Pterygoid fovea

J
3   Head of mandible - condylar process

K
4   Neck of mandible

L
5   Post. border of ramus of mandible

6   Ramus - vertical ramus

M
7   Angle of mandible

N
8   Oblique line

9   Inferior border

O
10 Body - horizontal ramus

P
11 Base

Q
12 Mental foramen

R
13 Mental tubercle - Gnathion

S
14 Mental protuberance

15 Alveolar bone surrounding teeth

T
16 Anterior border of ramus

U
17 Coronoid process - endocoronial ridge

V
18 Mandibular foramen

W
19 Lingula

20 Superior and inferior mental spines

X
21 Digastric fossa

Y
22 Mylohyoid line

Z
23 Mylohyoid groove

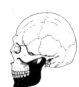

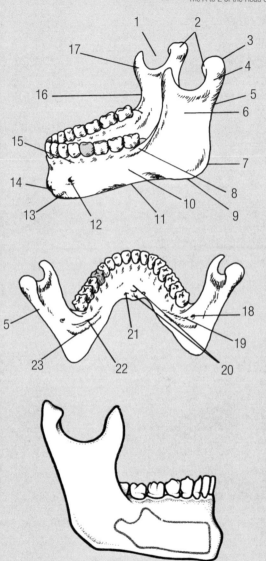

changes in the mandible from child <1yo to adult

F **Mandible**

B *Anterior*

C *radiology*
orthopantomogram = OPG

D
E *Used to show mandibular fractures and an overview of sinuses and complete dentition.*

F 1 Central incisor (21)*

G 2 Lateral incisor (22)

H 3 Canine (23)

I
J 4 First premolar (24)

K 5 Second premolar (25)

L 6 First molar (26)

M 7 Second molar (27)

N 8 Pulp chamber of molars (16, 17)

O 9 Coronoid process

P
Q 10 Head of mandible

R 11 Zygoma

S 12 Maxillary sinus

T 13 Anterior nasal spine of maxilla

U 14 Vomer (nasal septum)

V 15 Sites for the third molar (18, 28, 38, 48)

W 16 Hard palate

X
Y ** See Teeth overview page 114*

Z

96 © A. L. Neill

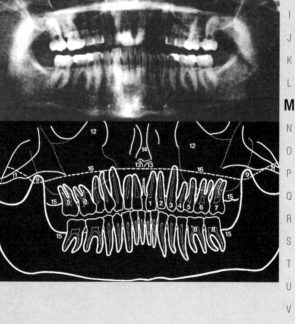

Mandible

Lateral

radiology
Showing relationship to surrounding soft tissue

1 Head of mandible – condylar process

2 Neck of the mandible

3 Hard palate

4 Soft palate

5 Anterior arch of the atlas (C1)

6 Odontoid process of the axis (C2) – dens

7 Posterior aspect of the tongue

8 Retropharyngeal sac

9 Epiglottis

10 Vallecula - fold anterior to epiglottis

11 Hyoid bone

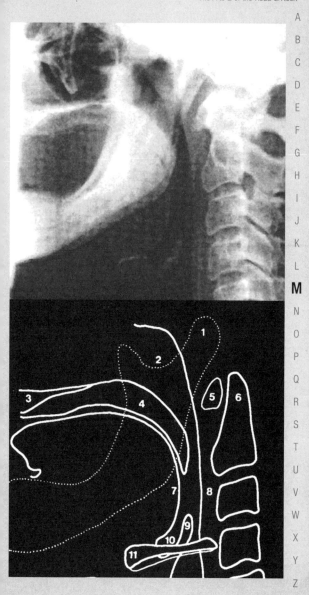

© A. L. Neill

Maxilla / Maxillae Bones

anterior / lateral / medial - see Palate for inferior view

(The Maxillae are 2 paired bones which form the dominant portion of the face and hold the upper teeth. The "overgrowth" of the Maxilla is often the reason for orthodontic treatment.)

1 Frontal process
2 Medial orbital surface
3 Infra-orbital margin
4 Zygomatic process
5 Infra-orbital foramen
6 Nasal notch
7 Nasal crest
8 Anterior nasal spine
9 Alveolar bone around teeth
10 Tuberosity / alveolar process
11 Infra-temporal surface
12 Orbital surface
13 Palatine process
14 Ethmoid crest
15 Canine jugun
16 Conchal crest
17 Naso-lacrimal process
18 *premaxillary suture is here - fuses with complete jaw growth*
Incisive canal *supported by the canine jugun*
19 Greater palatine canal - groove
20 Articulating surface – with palatine bones
21 Maxillary hiatus continues with the sinus
22 Nasal lacrimal groove

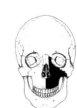

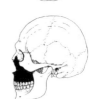

A
B
C
D
E
F
G
H
I
J
K
L
M
N
O
P
Q
R
S
T
U
V
W
X
Y
Z

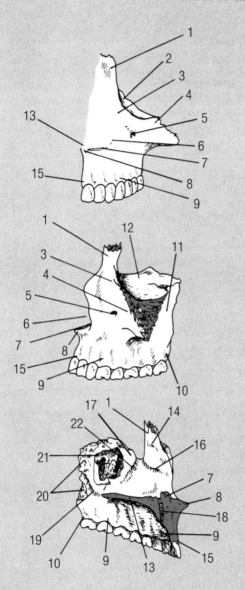

A
B
C
D
E
F
G
H
I
J
K
L
M
N
O
P
Q
R
S
T
U
V
W
X
Y
Z

A ## Nasal Bones and Cavity = NOSE

B *BONES external / internal / paired - posterior*

C The NOSE consists of: - 2 small thin rectangular bones below the
Glabella, the NASAL BONES; 2 lateral walls which house the 3 PAIRED
D TURBINATES or CONCHAE; the MEDIAL SEPTUM - made up of the
VOMER and the ETHMOID bones and the many cartilages which
E determine the length and shape of the nose and nasal nares (nostrils).

F The cavity is surrounded by sinuses which open into it and superiorly
by the Ethmoid plate allowing the OLFACTORY nerves to drop processes
G into the cavity. More details in the A-Z of Surface Anatomy.

Articulations:	with Frontal superiorly	All 2°
	with Lacrimal laterally with itself medially with Ethmoid inferiorly	fibrocartilagenous joints
SPECIAL FEATURES	"articulates" with nasal cartilages anteriorly	BS in septum does not extend to cartilage
superior & middle nasal conchae	parts of the Ethmoid bone	
inferior nasal conchae	2 small snail like bones lying on top of Palantine bones	

1 Frontal sinus
2 Nasal spine of frontal bone
2A Articulation with frontal bone
3 Nasal bone - external surface
3A Nasal bone internal surface
4 Perpendicular plate of ethmoid
5 Ant. nasal spine
6 Maxilla
6A Articulation b/n Nasal bones and Maxilla
7 Sphenoid bone - (pterygoid plates)
8 Vomer
9 Sphenoidal sinus
10 Crista Galli
11 Foramen for nasal vein
12 Notch for external nasal nerve
13 Articulation with other nasal bone
14 Lacrimal bone
15 Inferior concha and meatus
16 Palantine bone - perpendicular plate & incisive fossa
17 Sphenopalatine meatus
18 Superior concha and meatus
19 Middle concha and meatus

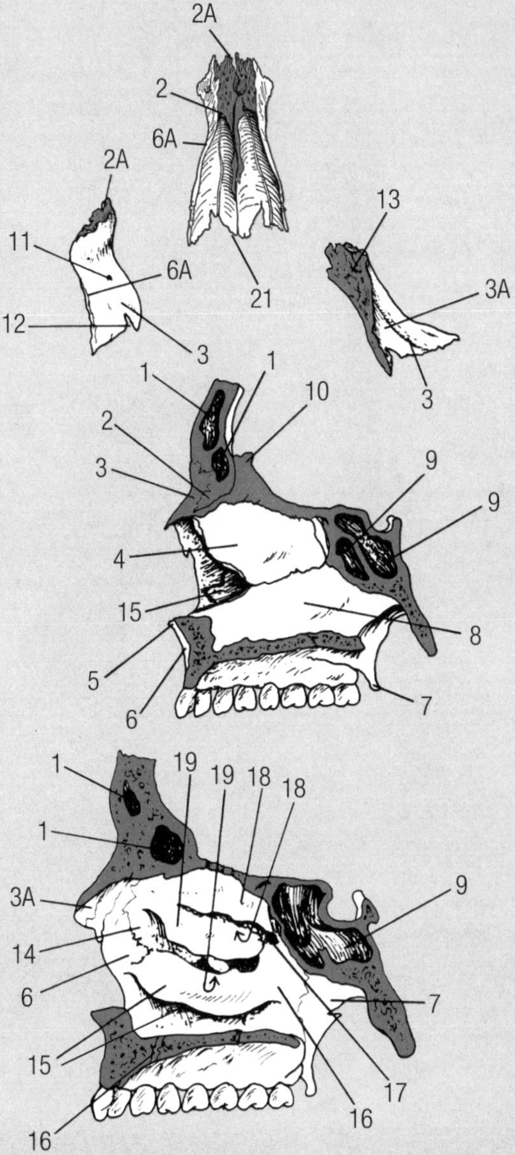
2A
2
6A
2A
11
6A
12
3
21
13
3A
3
1
1
10
2
3
9
9
4
15
8
5
6
7
1
19
19
18
18
1
3A
9
14
6
7
15
17
16
16

A Occipital bone *external / internal*

Articulations:	with Sphenoid	anteriorly
	with Vertebral Column	inferiorly
	with C1	laterally
	with C2	
Special features	large bowl-like bone with a hole at the infero-posterior portion of the skull	

1 Superior angle
2 Highest nuchal line
3 Superior nuchal line
4 Inferior nuchal line
5 Mastoid margin
6 Jugular process
7 Condylar fossa
8 Occipital condyle
9 Foramen magnum
10 Hypoglossal canal
11 Condylar canal
12 Lateral surface
13 Lateral angle
14 Occipital crest (internal)
15 Squamous surface
16 Occipital protuberance (internal)
17 Lambdoid margin
18 Groove for superior sagittal sinus
19 Posterior cerebral fossa / occipital fossa
20 Groove for transverse sinus
21 Attachment for tentorium cerebelli
22 Groove for sigmoid sinus
23 Jugluar notch
24 Jugular tubercle
25 Attachments for falx cerebri
26 Opisthion
27 Basion
28 Occipital sulcus - sagittal sinus

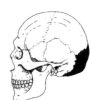
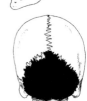

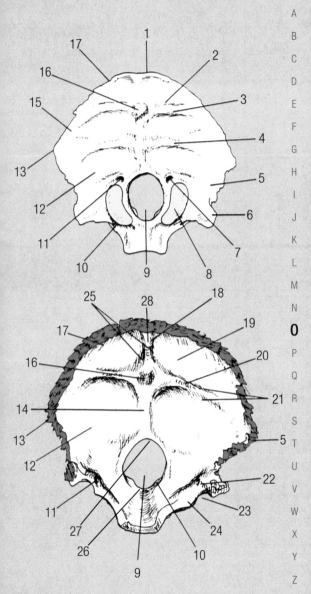

A Palate

B Inferior view - looking up into the palate - roof of the mouth

C Maxilla + Upper Teeth + Palatine bones

D 1 Nasopalatine NS emerging from the incisive
E   foramen (alveolare)

F 2 Greater palatine NS emerging from the greater
G   palatine foraminae

H 3 Lesser palatine NS emerging from the lessser
I   palatine foraminae

J 4 Hard palate

K 5 Soft palate

L 6 Nasal process

M

N

O

P

Q

R

S

T

U

V

W

X

Y

Z

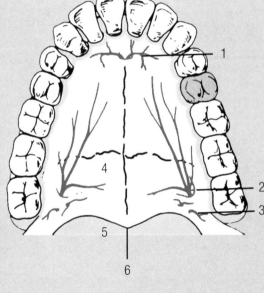

A **Palatine bones (Left)**

B *sagittal / medial / anterior / posterior*

Articulations:	mainly with the upper jaw (Maxilla) and the Sphenoid joints	2° fibrocartilagenous
Special features	L-shaped bones - forms the floor of the nasal cavity	

1 Perpendicular plate - vertical plate

2 Palato-maxillary suture

3 Maxilla

4 Orbital process

5 Spheno-palatine notch

6 Sphenoidal process -

6A Pterygo-palatine canal

7 Horizontal plane

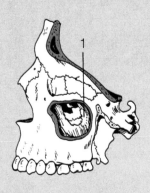

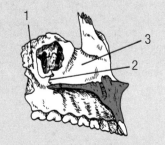

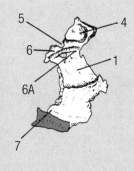

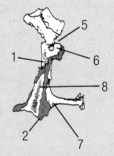

A **Parietal bone (Left)**

B *external / internal*

Articulations:	with the Frontal - anteriorly	All 2°
	with the Temporal - inferiorly with the Occipital - posteriorly with itself medially	fibro - cartilagenous joints
Special features	large square bone - largest of the cranial vault - even thickness all 4 corners make up the basis of the fontanelles in the infant	

1 Superior temporal line
2 Parietal eminence
3 Articulation with the occipital bone (lambdoid suture)
4 Articulation with the temporal bone (mastoid) parieto-mastoid suture
5 Articulation with the temporal (squamous) temporo-parietal suture
6 Articulation with the sphenoid (greater wing) spheno-parietal suture
7 Articulation with the frontal bone coronal suture
8 Inferior temporal line
9 Articulation between parietal bones sagittal suture
10 Frontal angle
11 Sphenoidal angle
12 Groove for frontal branch of middle meningeal vessels
13 Groove for parietal branch of middle meningeal vessels
14 Mastoid angle
15 Groove for sigmoid sinus
16 Occipital angle
17 Groove for superior sagittal sinus

A
B
C
D
E
F
G
H
I
J
K
L
M
N
O
P
Q
R
S
T
U
V
W
X
Y
Z

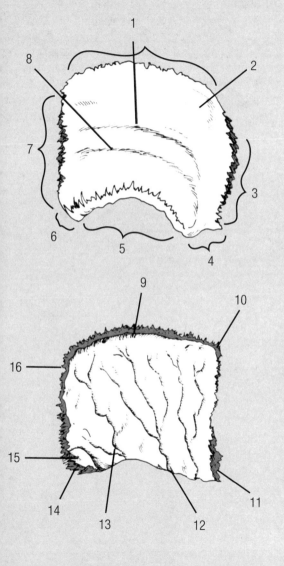

© A. L. Neill

Sphenoid

anterior / posterior / schema - development

A single wedge-shaped bone consisting of four parts: the central body; the lateral greater wings, the medial lesser wings and the lower pterygoid plates. The bone looks like a bat in flight and is the centre piece of the skull.

1 Articulation with L temporal bone
2 Orbital surface
3 Infratemporal crest
4 Body of the sphenoid
5 Openings for sphenoidal sinuses
6 Lesser wing (come across and meet to form jugum)
7 Squamosal suture - articulation with R Temporal bone
8 Superior orbital fissure
9 Foramen rotundum
10 Pterygoid canal
11 Rostrum
12 Vaginal process
13 Medial pterygoid plate
14 Pterygoid hamulus
15 Pterygoid notch
16 Lateral pterygoid plate
17 Pterygoid process
18 Sphenoid spine
19 Greater wing
19A Cerebral surface of the greater wing
20 Anterior clinoid process
21 Posterior clinoid process
22 Dorsum sellae
23 Articulation with occiput

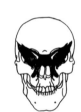

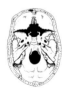

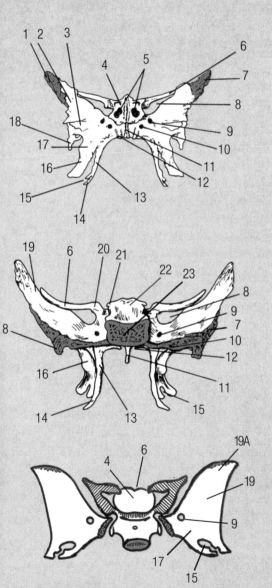

Teeth *Overview*

There are many different methods used to name teeth, define their positions and dentitions and describe their surfaces. This overview shows the 1o & 2o dentitions, describes their positions and tooth types using some of the better known methods.

Teeth are labeled XY on the Left and Right - X is the quadrant of the teeth and dentition type - adult or child - Y is the tooth type (devised by the Federation Dentaire Internationale).

1 Maxillary upper right quadrant - adult
2 Maxillary upper left quadrant - adult
3 Mandibular lower left quadrant - adult
4 Mandibular lower right quadrant - adult
5 Maxillary upper right quadrant - child
6 Maxillary upper left quadrant - child
7 Mandibular lower left quadrant - child
8 Mandibular lower right quadrant - child

1 Central Incisor
2 Lateral Incisor
3 Canine
4 First Pre-molar
5 Second Pre-molar
6 First Molar
7 Second Molar
8 Third Molar

A Palatal - upper tooth surface facing the inside of the mouth
B Buccal - any tooth surface facing the cheek
C Mesial - any tooth more anterior than the 1st molar
D Distal - all teeth behind the 1st molar
E Lingual - lower tooth surface facing the tongue
F Occlusal - any tooth surface which abuts with another tooth-bite surface (shown surface)
G Labial - any tooth surface facing the lips

© A. L. Neill

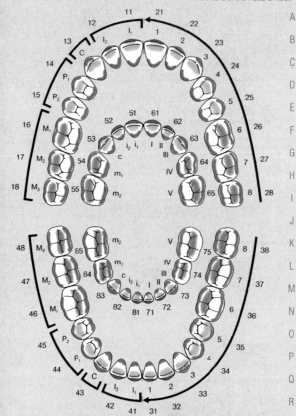

Teeth are labeled by letters and subscripts on the Right letters

I = incisors $2°$ dention (adult) i = incisors $1°$ dentition (child)

C = canine c = canine

M = molar m = molar

P = premolar

Teeth are labeled using roman numerals in the smaller circle to demonstrate this method - (not commonly used)

Each tooth has several surfaces and lies in different oral regions

A **Temporal bone (Left)** *external / inferior / internal*

B *Temporal = TIME. This bone shows first signs of aging - grey hair. It is
involved in both the wall and the base of the skull. Temporal bones contain
C the auditory ossicles/ear bones & form the only joint with the mandible.*

D 1 Suprameatal triangle
2 Groove for middle temporal artery
E 3 Parietal notch
4 Squamo-mastoid suture
F 5 Mastoid area
6 Mastoid process
G 7 Sheath of styloid process
8 Styloid process
H 9 Tympanic part I
10 External acoustic meatus / anterior border (bony ear hole)
I 11 Tympanosquamosal (squamotympanic) fissure
12 Mandibular fossa
J 13 Zygomatic process
14 Articular tubercle
K 15 Postglenoid tubercle
16 Squamous part - squama
L 17 Stylomastoid foramen
18 Mastoid notch - digastric groove
M 19 Occipital groove
20 Jugular surface
N 21 Jugular fossa
22 Canaliculus (opening) for tympanic nerve
O 23 Petrous part
24 Carotid canal
P 25 Edge of tegmen tympani
26 Groove for the middle meningeal vessels
Q 27 Groove for the superior petrosal sinus
R 28 Articulation with the greater wing of the sphenoid
spheno-temporal suture
U 29 Zygomatic process
30 Groove for the middle meningeal vessels
V 31 Internal acoustic meatus
32 Articulates with the occipital bone
W 33 Aqueduct of the vestibule
34 Mastoid foramen
X 35 Groove for sigmoid sinus - sigmoid sulcus
36 Arcuate eminence
Y 37 Articulates with the parietal bone temporoparietal suture
Z

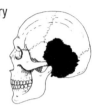

© A. L. Neill

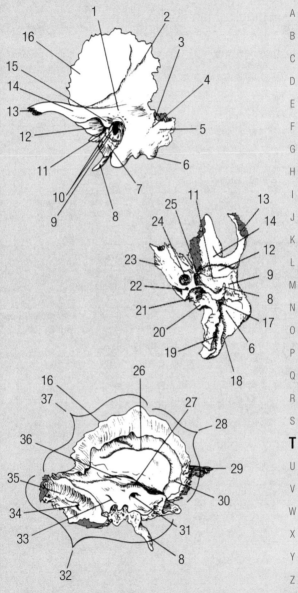

A **Temporo-Mandibular Joint = TMJ**

B *closed - lateral / medial*

C *open - sagittal*

D *(only SYNOVIAL joint in the skull).*

E **BS** *superficial temporal & maxillary arteries*

F **NS** *auriculotemporal & masseteric branches of mandibular*
G *branch of Trigeminal N (CN5)*

H **A** *depression/elevation, protrusion/retraction,*
lateral movements

I

1 Fibrous capsule

J 2 Lateral TMJ lig

K 3 Stylomandibular lig

L 4 Mandible

M 5 Ant. Temporal attachment of meniscus

N 6 Meniscus

O 7 Ant. mandibular attachment

P 8 Condyle of mandible

Q 9 Posterior attachment

10 Sphenomandibular lig

R 11 Posterior temporal attachment

S 12 Lower joint compartment

T 13 Temporal bone

U 14 Upper compartment

V 15 Ext. auditory meatus

W

X

Y

Z

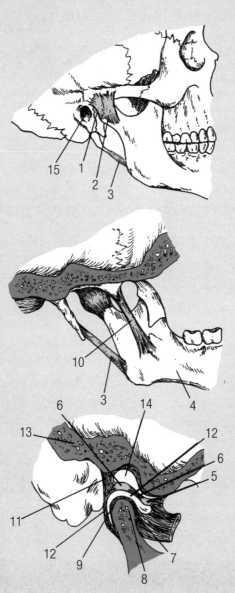

A # **Temporo-Mandibular Joint (TMJ)** *Lateral*

B *radiology*

C *Open - upper*
Shut - lower

D 1 Head of mandible – condylar process

E 2 Neck of the mandible

F 3 Coronoid process

G 4 Zygomatic arch

H 5 External auditory meatus + handle of the malleus

I 6 Articular cubicle

J 7 Tympanic plate

K 8 Mastoid process

L 9 Groove for posterior belly of digastric muscle

L 10 Mandibular fossa

M 11 Greater wing of the sphenoid (basal surface)

N 12 Lesser wing of the sphenoid

O

P

Q

R

S

T

U

V

W

X

Y

Z

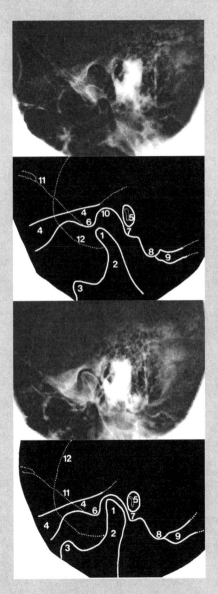

Vertebrae *Typical cervical C3-7*

superior

Articulations:	with vertebra above & below -2 unpaired joints 2 paired joints	VB -VB joints symphysis Spinous process joints syndesmosis paired zygapophyseal planar synovial paired TP joints fibrous sydesmosis
Special features	transverse foramen bifid spinous process small curved bodies	

1 Body
2 Pedicle
3 Superior articular facet
4 Vertebral foramen
5 Lamina
6 Spinous process - bifid*
7 Post. tubercle of TP
8 Transverse foramen*
9 Sulcus for peripheral N outlet
10 Anterior tubercle of TP

*only in cervical vertebrae

122

© A. L. Neill

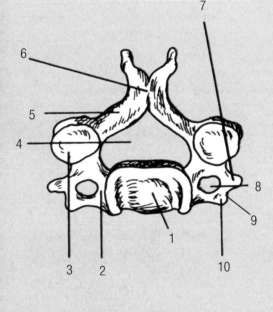

A **Vomer**

B *lateral / posterior / in situ*

C *A single small narrow frail plough-shaped midline bone. It is the*
D *deviation of this bone which may obstruct the nasal airways.*

E

1 Ala (Alae)

F
2 Articulation with maxillae and palatine
maxillovomer suture / palatinovomer suture

G
3 Groove for the nasopalantine nerves and vessels

H
4 Articulation with nasal cartilages

I
5 Articulation with sphenoid bone

J
6 Articulation with the ethmoid plate

K
7 Perpendicular plate of the Ethmoid

8 Body of vomer

L
9 Maxillae areolar bone

M
10 Medial pterygoid plate

N
11 Frontal bone

O
12 Sphenoid sinus

P
13 Anterior of nasal bones

Q
14 Frontal sinus

R

S

T

U

V

W

X

Y

Z

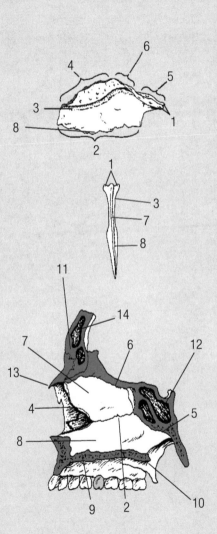

A **Zygoma = CHEEK BONES**

B *antero-lateral / postero-medial*

C *These bones form the prominent corners of the face under the orbital rim.*

D 1 Frontal process

E 2 Zygomatico-facial formina

F 3 Articulation with the frontal bone

G 4 Articulation with the sphenoid

5 Zygomatico-orbital foramina

H 6 Articulation with maxilla

I 7 Zyomatico-temporal foramina

J 8 Temporal process

K 9 Maxillary process

L 10 Orbital surface

M

N

O

P

Q

R

S

T

U

V

W

X

Y

Z

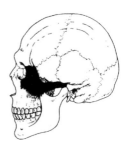

© A. L. Neill

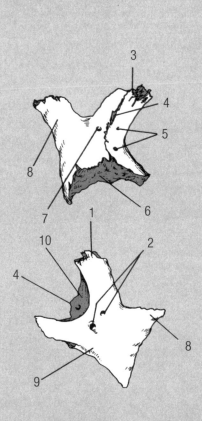

MUSCLES OF THE HEAD & NECK

MUSCLES OF THE HEAD & NECK regional & functional guide

■ Muscles of caput/basocranium and cervical spine

■ Muscles of expression

■ **Muscles of the eye and ear**

■ Muscles of mastication

■ Muscles of the hyoid and thyroid / anterior triangle

■ Muscles of pharynx and larynx

■ **Muscles of the tongue**

Index of Muscles

L

Lateral Cricoarytenoid
Lateral Pterygoid *see also Pterygoids*
Lateral Rectus
Levator Anguli Oris (Caninus)
Levator Labii Superioris
Levator Labii Superioris Alaeque Nasi
Levator Palpebrae Superioris
Levator Veli Palatini
Linguali muscles = Intrinsic muscles of the Tongue
Longissimus Capitus
Longissimus Cervicis
Longus Capitus
Longus Colli

M

Masseter
Medial Pterygoid *see also Pterygoids*
Medial Rectus
Mentalis
Multifidus Cervicis
Muscularis Uvulae
Mylohyoid

N

Nasalis

O

Oblique Arytenoid *see Arytenoids*
Obliquis Capitis Inferior
Obliquis Capitis Superior
Occipitalis *see Epicranius*
Occipitofrontalis *see Epicranius*
Omohyoid
Orbicularis Oculi
Orbicularis Oris

P Q

Palatoglossus
Palatopharyngeus
Pharyngeal Constrictors - inferior
Pharyngeal Constrictors - middle
Pharyngeal Constrictors - superior
Platysma
Posterior Cricoarytenoid
Procerus
Pterygoids *see also Lateral & Medial Pterygoids*

R

Rectus Capitus Anterior
Rectus Capitus Lateralis
Rectus Capitus Posterior Major
Rectus Capitus Posterior Minor
Risorius
Rotatores-Longus and Brevis (Cervical region)

S

Salpingopharyngeus
Scalenus Anterior
Scalenus Medius
Scalenus Minimus
Scalenus Posterior
Semispinalis Capitus, Cervicis
Sphincter Pupillae *see Pupillary muscles*
Splenius Capitus
Splenius Cervicus
Stapedius
Sternocleidomastoid
Sternohyoid
Sternothyroid
Styloglossus
Stylohyoid
Stylopharyngeus
Superior Lingualis *see Linguali muscles/Intrinsic muscles of the Tongue*
Superior Oblique
Superior Rectus

T

Temporalis
Temporoparietalis
Tensor Tympani
Tensor Veli Palatini
Thyroarytenoid
Thyroepiglotticus
Thyrohyoid
Transverse Arytenoid *see Arytenoids*
Transverse Lingualis *see Linguali muscles/Intrinsic muscles of the Tongue*

UV

Uvulae Muscularis aka Muscularis Uvulae
Vocalis *see also Thyroarytenoid*

WXYZ

Zygomaticus Major
Zygomaticus Minor

Classification of Muscles

There are three types of muscle tissue and this book discusses only one of them - SKELETAL MUSCLE. The other two are smooth muscle (for the gut and other areas of involuntary movement) and cardiac muscle (for the heart).

SKELETAL muscle is defined as muscle which is "striated" or striped, indicating an ordered cell structure, of myosin and actin filaments, and is generally under voluntary control, which has an action on the skeleton or bones in the body.

In its relaxed form it is at its maximum length and this is generally how the tissue is found. Stimulation generally causes contraction and a shortening and thickening of the tissue. As it is attached to a minimum of two points, the Origin (O) and the insertion (I) - although these may be arbitrarily named – this "contraction" brings these two points closer together. To reverse this, another muscle must be attached to two different points which when they move together cause a reversal of the position of the two or more affected bones, hence for each muscle there is an antagonist (opposing muscle) and in many situations a synergist (a muscle which enhances the original movement).

There are a few exceptions to this. For example SPHINCTERS are circular groups of muscle fibres which upon contraction close the circle they have formed and may not be attached to bones at all. Their function is to prevent leakage or passage of material from one area to another.

Many of the MUSCLES OF FACIAL EXPRESSION are inserted into the deep fascia of the skin and hence change the soft tissues of the face but do not affect the bones underneath. We as humans have a great deal of these muscles, and they may be shifted or injured in many cosmetic procedures because of this structure.

Muscle are shaped to allow their contraction to occur in the most efficient manner, for example sheets of muscles cover expanses of tissue to contain them, as in the OBLIQUES to contain and move bulky abdominal contents, or DIAPHRAGMS to separate as well as move large anatomical regions around, while TERES muscles are small, cordlike, focused groups of fibres for very specific movements.

Generally the smaller the muscles, the deeper they are placed, so larger and more powerful muscles can cover them, for example ZYGOMATICUS MAJOR covers ZYGOMATICUS MINOR. Smaller muscles generally have more specific actions, are more resilient but weaker, they contract and relax repeatedly for example, to maintain position of the face, as in the small muscles around the nose and upper lips of the face. They are essential for a "balanced" even facial expression and lip movement and can be affected greatly in cosmetic surgery and increasingly injected procedures. Larger, longer muscles by definition cannot be as precise but have larger ranges of motion and more power and are placed more superficially - closer to the surface, as in ERECTOR SPINAE.

Fibrous tissue inserts give the muscle more strength but less ability to move, as in RECTUS ABDOMINUS versus TRAPEZIUS, but it is these large surface/superficial muscles whose shape can be changed and defined by gross movement exercises.

Muscles are named using many different criteria singly or in combination: for example they may be named according to their action –Supinator, Pronator and size – Adductor Magnus, Adductor Longus, Adductor Brevis; their shape and location- Biceps Brachii, Triceps Brachii, Quadratus Lumborum, Interossei, Intercostals; the direction of their muscle fibres and anatomical layer– Obliquus Externus Abdominus, Obliquus Internus Abdominus and there does not seem to be a consistent pattern in this naming - only that from the name it is often possible to determine their site, action &/or shape and this helps when memorizing these muscles.

Between each muscle group is a fascial layer to transport in the BVs and the Nerves. This is particularly important in the Head & Neck because of the great mobility in this region.

Testing of a muscle is often impossible to do singly and they must be tested as an anatomical and functional group. The tests are generally graded 1-5, with 5 being the strongest and 3 being the point where when appropriate the muscle can overcome Gravity, often a natural form of resistance to the muscle action. This level of testing muscles is not dealt with in this book and will be discussed in the *A to Z of Muscle and Sensory testing* to follow - it is also examined in some detail in the *A to Z of Peripheral Nerves* - however testing of the primary action of most muscles is listed on each page as a guide to the practitioner for basic testing and grouping of muscles. Please use this testing section as a guide only.

Examination of structures in the Head and Neck in general and an overview of the area have been included in the front of the book.

Muscles of the Eye

Note all 6 of these muscles act "in concert" in eye movement and depend upon the fixation and focus of the eye, included is the muscle which moves the eyelid to follow the eye gaze, hence 6+1.

Extrinsic

Muscles responsible for movement of the upper eyelid

1 Levator Palpebrae Superioris
NS oculomotor N (CN III)
BS supraorbital, branches of ophthalmic N (from CN V_1)

Muscles responsible for movement of the eyeball

2 Recti muscles - Inferior/Superior, Medial/Lateral.
These muscles are straight and are responsible for one movement up/down, in/out

3 Oblique muscles - Inferior, Superior
These muscles are attached via a trochlea 3t or pulley and movements therefore vary on eye position and are diagonal up and out/ down and in

All are attached to the scleral surface, the Recti via the optic canal on the common annular tendon, (5) & the Obliques via bones in the optic cavity (6)

NS oculomotor N (CNIII) - except Lateral Rectus - abducent N (CN VI) (CNVI) and Superior Oblique - trochlea N (CN IV)
BS ophthalmic and branches of internal carotid

Note the CN responsible for vision is the Optic N CN II (8) which exits from the back of the pupil through the optic canal

Intrinsic

These muscles are responsible for moving structures within the eyeball and are not shown but affect the lens (9) and iris (7).

NS Oculomotor N (CN III) parasympathetic outflow
BS ophthalmic and branches of internal carotid

10 Ciliaris
11 Dilator Pupillae
12 Sphincter Pupillae

The cornea (13) is a modified form of the CT which forms the sclera and the ciliary body (14) attaches long strands of connecting fibres (15) which affect the curvature of the lens.

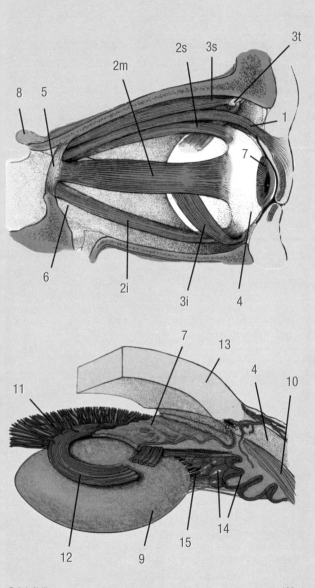

Muscles of the Eye
in situ
removal of superficial tissue / coronal section / enucleation with muscle bed intact

1 Levator palpebrae superioris
2 4 x recti muscles (superior, inferior, lateral, medial)
3 2 x oblique muscles (superior, inferior)
4 Trochlear N (CN IV)
5 Ciliary ganglion (CN III)
6 Abducens N (CN VI)
7 Oculomotor N + branches (CN III)
8 Trochlea
9 Superior orbital notch
10 Superior orbital fissure
11 Optic N (CN II)
12 Lacrimal gland

see orbital cavity for bony orbit P48

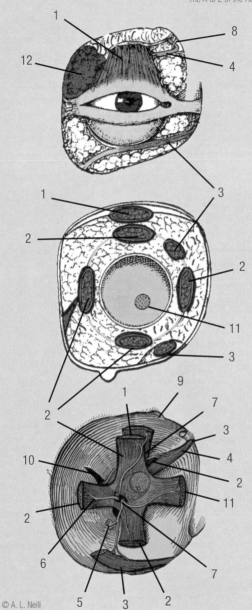

A B

Face – muscles of expression and lip and cheek movement

C *Anterior – major muscles of the face*

D 1 Frontalis muscle belly

E 2 Temporalis

F 3 muscles of the nose
c = Compressor naris
G d = Dilator naris
H s = Depressor septi nasi

I 4 4L Levator anguli oris
4D Depressor anguli oris

J

K 5 Masseter

6 Buccinator

L 7 Risorius

M 8 Orbicularis oris

N 9 Depressor labii inferioris

O 10 Mentalis

11 Platysma – on both the lower face & neck

P 12 split in the Platysma may widen with age leading to softening and heaviness of the jawline sagging of the chin skin

Q

R

13 Zygomaticus M = Major, m = minor

S 14 Levator labii superioris
n = Levator labii superioris alaeque nasi

T

U 15 Orbicularis oculi

V 16 Depressor supercili

W 17 Corrugator

X 18 Procerus

Y 19 Epicranius = Frontalis + Galea aponeurosis + Occipitalis (not seen)

Z

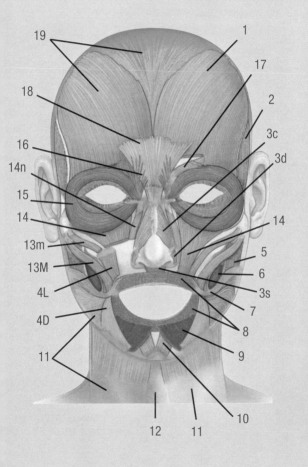

Muscles of the Face – Expression

Anterolateral view

These muscles are often involved in cosmetic surgery and their function may be compromised by incisions at the level of the deep fascia.

1 Buccinator

2 Corrugator supercili

3 Depressor anguli Oris -

4 Depressor labii inferioris

(4) Incisivus labii inferioris deeper

5 Depressor septi

6 Occipitofrontalis - a - Frontalis p - Occipitalis

7 Levator anguli oris (caninus),

8 Levator labii superioris

(8) Incisivus labii superioris deeper

9 Levator labii superioris alaeque nasi
   also (overlying Incisivus sup.)

10 Mentalis

11 Nasalis (compressor & dilator)

12 Orbicularis oculi

13 Orbicularis oris

14 Platysma

15 Procerus

16 Risorius

17 Zygomaticus major

18 Zygomaticus minor

NS   facial N (CN VII)
BS   facial

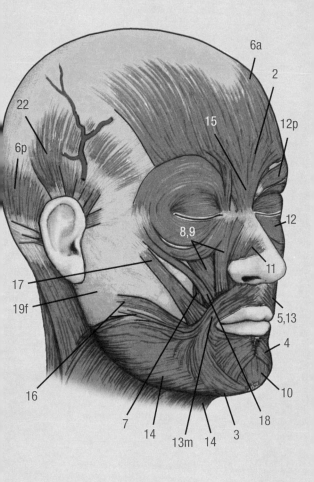

Mastication *Coronal section posterior view*

Primary movers of the Mandible + chewing and initiation of swallowing

Muscles of mastication are all attached to the Mandible (Jaw bone) and are part of the Splanchnocranium. Those initiating swallowing move the food to the back of the throat and then into the oropharynx

19 Masseter (F = Fascia)

20 Pterygoids Lateral (deep to Masseter)

21 Pterygoids Medial (deep to Buccinator)

22 Temporalis

All are attached to the Mandible – Jaw bone and part of the Splanchnocranium

NS trigeminal N –mandibular branch (CN V$_3$)
BS trigeminal and facial branches

Articulation & Swallowing *See also muscles of the Hyoid*

Primarily involved in speech and initiation of swallowing but have other functions in expression. They are often involved in "Stroke" patients affecting both speech and eating.

31 Genioglossus

32 Geniohyoid

33 Styloglossus*

34 Hypoglossus

35 Stylohyoid*

36 Thyrohyoid*

37 Sternohyoid*

38 Sternothyroid*

39 Mylohyoid

40 Digastric*

NS hypoglossal (CN XII) and C1-3 of ansa cervicalis
BS facial branches

50 Mandibular sling = insertion raphe

51 Mandibular condyle

52 Interarticular disc of the TMJ

53 Sphenoid

See Muscles of the Hyoid and Thyroid

22
20
53
52
51

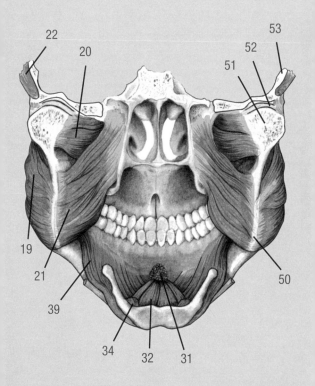

19
21
39
34
32
31
50

Muscles of the Hyoid bone & Thyroid cartilage (Larynx)

The Hyoid bone and the Larynx hang b/n the SUPRA-HYOID and INFRAHYOID muscles

They move with swallowing, breathing and speech

SWALLOWING cannot commence w/o the Mandible being fixed

It cannot continue w/o the Sternum and Clavicle being fixed to allow for the Hyoid to be depressed

Arrows show the directions of the muscles

These muscles determine the chin line and are involved in cosmetic surgery – Several muscles rely on tendinous slings and have two bellies to function.

Elevator Muscles

1. Palatoglossus
2. Stylopharyngeus
3. Thyrohyoid
4. Pharyngeal constrictors
5. Stylohyoid
6. Geniohyoid
7. Digastric
8. Mylohyoid

Depressor Muscles

9. Sternohyoid
10. Omohyoid
11. Sternothyroid
3. Thyrohyoid (both functions)

NS ansa cervicalis C1-3
BS facial and thyroid vessels

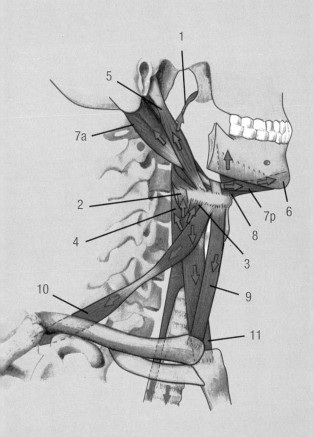

A

Muscles of the Neck

B

NECK – has 2 major groups of muscles

1 those concerned with the neck movement
C
i.e. movement of the cervical spine & head
2 those concerned with the anterior neck structures i.e. the larynx & pharynx.

D

Group 1

E

deep posterior - suboccipital muscles – extensors / hyperextensors/rotators and stabilizers

F

Rectus Capitus Posterior – Major and Minor
G
Obliquuis Capitus muscles
Cervical & Cephalic / Capitus regions of the muscles of the VC (5, 6)
H **NS** segmental - dorsal rami of the related SNs
BS dorsal branches of the carotids

I

deep anterior - prevertebral flexors, rotators and stabilizers

J

Rectus Capitus ant. & lat. (1, 10)
Longus Colli supporting mainly the cervical vertebrae (8) and
K
Longus Capitus (9) supporting mainly the head
NS segmental - ventral rami of related SNs
L **BS** branches of carotids and other local vessels

M These muscles are covered by the prevertebral fascia of the neck.

anterior - flexors, rotators

N

Scalenii muscles -anterior, medial and posterior (7)
NS segmental anterior branches of the ventral rami
O
BS superficial cervical

P These muscles are covered by the prevertebral fascia of the neck.

Q 1 Rectus capitus lateralis
2 Splenius capitus
R 3 Digastricus – post belly
4 Levator scapulae
S 5 Longissimus cervicus
6 Iliocostalis cervicus
T 7 Scalenes a = ant , m = middle p = post
8 Longus colli
U 9 Longus capitus
10 Rectus capitus anterior
V 11 Mastoid and styloid processes
12 Ribs 1 & 2
W 13 ALL
14 Sphenoid
X 15 EAM
16 Occiput
Y

Z

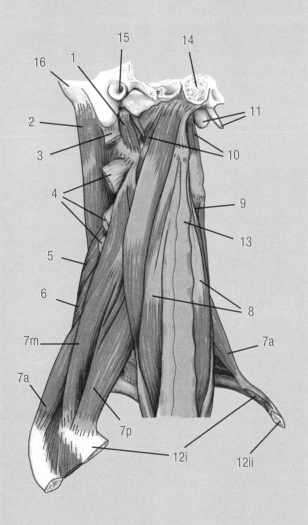

Muscles of the Pharynx

Lateral

Defn: the space b/n the mouth and oesophagus – a modified muscular tube directing the food bolus to the GIT.

Lifting the Pharynx closes the auditory tube and nasopharynx (10, 11) food moves to the back of the throat – swallowing begins coordinated by the constrictors (1). It is supported by ligs (3, 12) & muscles (2).

BS   facial, maxillary
NS   CN X – vagus, branches of ansa cervicalis (C1-3)

1 Pharyngeal constrictors
    i = inferior
    m = middle
    s = superior

2 Stylopharyngeus

3 Stylohyoid lig

4 Thyroid cartilage

5 Thyrohyoid membrane

6 Hyoid bone

7 Mylohyoid muscle

8 Mandible

9 Buccinator

10 Palatopharyngeus

11 Salpingopharyngeus

12 Cricothyroid

13 Oesophagus

14 Trachea

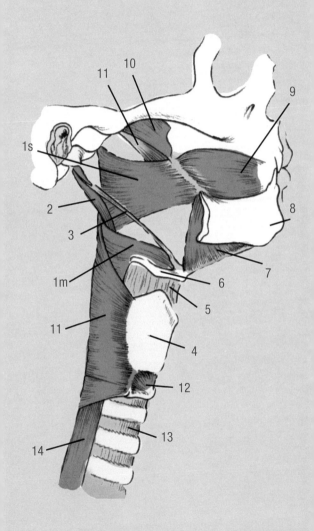

A Aryepiglotticus

part of the muscles of the Larynx

O apex of the arytenoid cartilage

I lateral border of epiglottus

A aids in the closure of the opening of the larynx (additis) moves the arytenoids to the epiglottic tubercle

NS recurrent laryngeal N (branch of vagus CN X)

BS laryngeal and thyroid vessels

B C D E F G H I J K L M N O P Q R S T U V W X Y Z

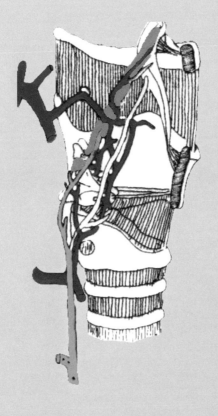

A Arytenoids

B *Oblique, Transverse -see also Cricoarytenoids*

C *part of the muscles of the Larynx*
Involved in the pitch of the voice and breathing

D
Posterior – trachea cut away

E

F *Oblique*

O/I b/n the muscular processes of the arytenoid cartilages

G **A** adduction of the aryepiglottic fold and the vocal cords to cause closure
with aryepiglotticus forms a sphincter of the laryngeal outlet

H **NS** recurrent laryngeal N (branch of vagus CN X)

I **BS** laryngeal and thyroid vessels

J *Transverse*

K **O/I** b/n the muscular processes of the arytenoid cartilages - medial on one
to the posterior surface of the other

L **A** adduction of the arytenoid cartilages & attached vocal cords - closure
of the rima glottis

M **NS** recurrent laryngeal N (branch of vagus CN X)

BS laryngeal and thyroid vessels

N

O 1 Hyoid

P 2 Epiglottis

Q 3 Aryepiglottis

R 4 Oblique arytenoid

S 5 Transverse arytenoid

6 Cricoid cartilage

T 7 Thyroid gland (outline)

U 8 Trachea

V 9 Arytenoid cartilage

W *Note the larynx is normally closed - antagonistic muscular contraction forces*

X *the structure open, hence in paralysis the larynx will close and prevent*
the passage of air

Y

Z

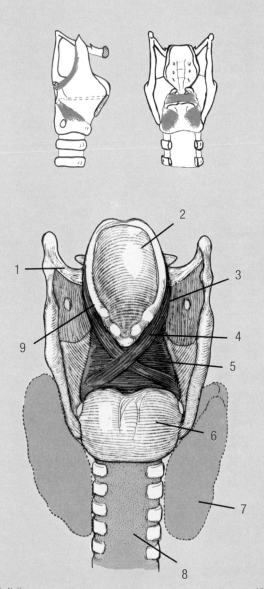

A Auricularis

anterior, posterior, superior

Extrinsic muscles of the Ear (present in 30%)

O ant. epicranial aponeurosis
post. mastoid process of temporalis
sup. epicranial aponeurosis

I ant. root of auricle
post. root of auricle
sup. root of auricle

A moves ear pinna

NS facial N (CN VII)

BS facial / temporal

T present if there is movement of the ear

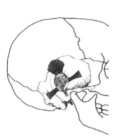

© A. L. Neill

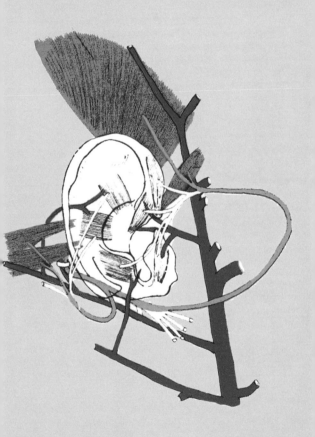

A **Buccinator**

B *part of the muscles of mastication*

C **O** lateral – outer surface of alveolar process of Maxilla
lateral surface (mandible)

D **I** deep part of the orbicularis oris deep fascia of the face
with aryepiglotticus forms a sphincter of the laryngeal outlet

E **A** compresses cheeks against the teeth - draws the angle of the
mouth down and laterally

F
NS facial N (CN VII)

G **BS** facial and maxillary
T ability to blow a saxophone or shape lips in this way

H

I

J

K

L

M

N

O

P

Q

R

S

T

U

V

W

X

Y

Z

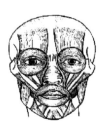

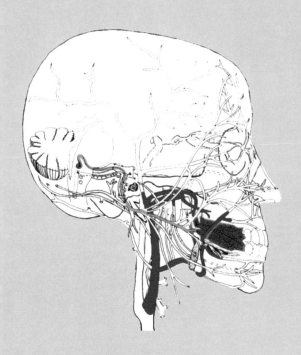

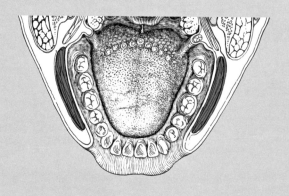

A **Ciliaris**

B *part of the muscles of the Eye*

C 0   scleral spur

I   stroma of the choroid

with aryepiglotticus forms a sphincter of the laryngeal outlet

A   modify the shape of the lens for distant (thinning of the
lens – less convexity) or close focus (thickening of the
lens – increased convexity)

NS   oculomotor (CN III) parasympathetic fibres - for near focus -
superior cervical ganglion - long ciliary Ns - for far vision

BS   lacrimal and ophthalmic branches of internal carotid

T   ability to focus *(note: other factors are relevant but the loss of
elasticity of the lens and the muscle to contract effectively contribute
to changes in vision)*

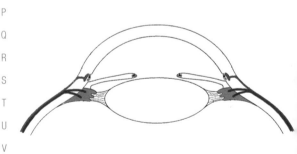

© A. L. Neill

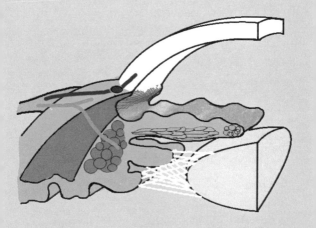

A Corrugator Supercili

B *part of the muscles of facial expression*

C **O** medial suprorbital margin (Frontal bone)
I deep fascia of the skin in the midpart of the orbital arch - glabella
D **A** pulls brows down and medially, frowning
NS facial N, supraorbital supratrochlear branches (CN VII)
E **BS** facial, ophthalmic
T ability to wrinkle brow as in frowning

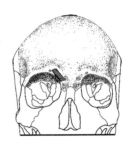

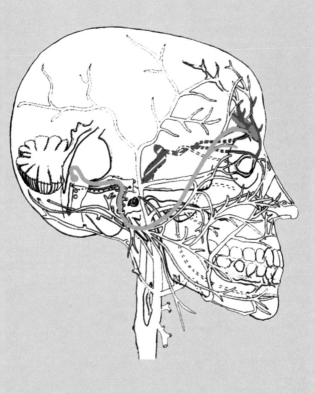

A # Cricoarytenoids

B *Superior – part of the muscles of the Larynx*

C *Involved in the pitch of the voice*

D ## Posterior

E
- **0** posterior horn of the arytenoids cartilages
- **I** posterior nodule of the Cricoid cartilage
F
- **NS** recurrent laryngeal N (CNX)
- **BS** laryngeal and thyroid vessels

G ## Transverse

H
- **0** posterior horn of the arytenoids cartilages
I
- **I** lateral walls of the Cricoid cartilage
- **NS** recurrent laryngeal N (CNX)
J
- **BS** laryngeal and thyroid vessels
- **T** test eye movements
K

L 1 Transverse cricoarytenoid

M 2 Posterior cricoarytenoid

N 3 Cricoid cartilage

O 4 Thyroid cartilage

P

Q

R

S

T

U

V

W

X

Y

Z

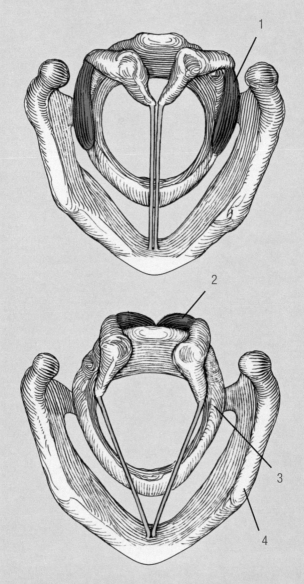

A

Cricothyroid

B *part of the muscles of the Larynx*

C **O** anterolateral aspect of the cricoid cartilage

I inferior cornu and lower lamina of the thyroid cartilage

D **A** tilts thyroid cartilage forwards, lengthening & tightening the vocal cords

NS superior laryngeal N (branch of the vagus N = CN X)

E **BS** cricothyroid branches of superior and inferior thyroid arteries

F **T** ability to change voice pitch and tone

G

H

I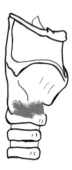

J

K

L

M

N

O

P

Q

R

S

T

U

V

W

X

Y

Z

© A. L. Neill

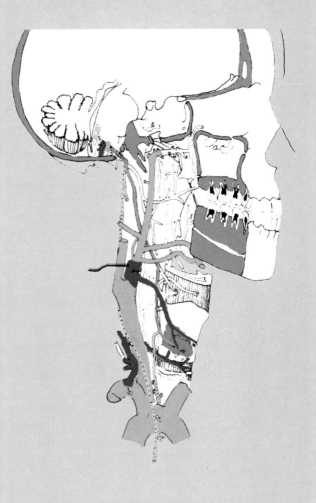

Depressors

part of the muscles of facial expression

Depressor Anguli Oris

O oblique lines (mandible) below and lateral to labii inferioris

D I deep fascia - at the corner of the lips - interdigitating other facial muscles

A turns the corners of the lips down as in frowning

NS facial N, maxillary branch (CN VII)

BS facial - mandibular + inferior labial branches

T ability to turn the corners of the mouth down as in frowning

Depressor Labii Inferioris

O anterior-medial surfaces of mandible

I deep fascia medial to the corners of the lips

A pulls lips down and back (with platysma)

NS facial N, superior buccal & mandibular branches (CN VII)

BS facial – inferior labial branches + inferior alveolar

T ability to draw back lips and tighten neck (continuous with platysma)

Depressor Septi

O anterior-medial surfaces of maxilla (incisive fossa)

I deep fascia at the base of the nose

A pulls nostrils inwards and lips up

NS facial N, maxillary branch (CN VII)

BS facial -maxillary, superior buccal branches

T ability to constrict nostrils (difficult to detect)

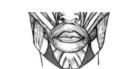

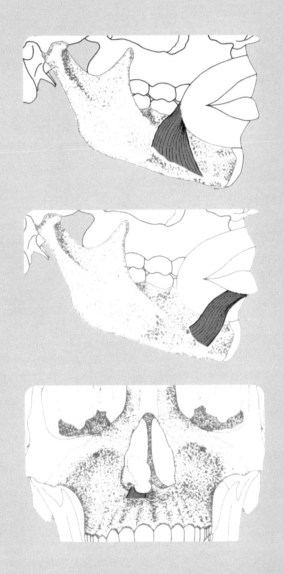

A

Digastricus

B

Digastric muscle

C

part of the muscles of the Hyoid (anterior neck) 2 muscular bellies anterior / posterior passing through a fibrous loop

D **O** anterior - inner side (lingular) of jaw (mandible)

E posterior - mastoid notch (temporal bone)

I slides through the hyoid tendon/ligamentous loop

F **A** elevates, retracts and protracts hyoid

depresses mandible

G **NS** anterior - trigeminal N (CN V) - mylohyoid branch

posterior - facial N (CN VII)

H **BS** facial mandibular branch

superior cervical

I

T open jaw against R

J note movement of hyoid on swallowing

K

L

M

N

O

P

Q

R

S

T

U

V

W

X

Y

Z

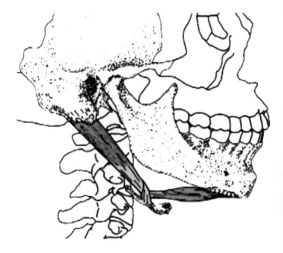

© A. L. Neill

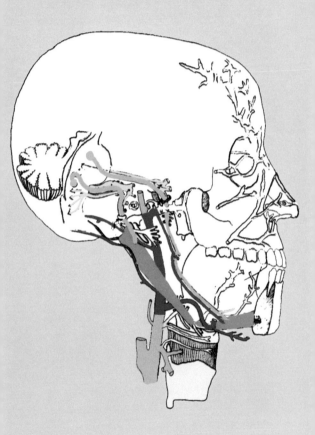

A # Epicranius

B *Frontalis + Occipitalis = Occipito-Frontalis*

C *Galea Aponeurosis = fibrous connection b/n the 2 muscle "bellies"*

D *2 heads anterior = Frontalis*

E *posterior = Occipitalis*

F ## Frontalis

G **O** skull aponeurosis
  I superficial fascia superior to brow
H **A** raises eyebrows / wrinkles forehead
  NS facial N temporal branches (CN VII)
I **BS** supraorbital supratrochlear branches of ophthalmic artery

J ## Occipitalis

K **O** Occipital bone - mastoid process (temporalis)
  I skull aponeurosis
L **A** draws scalp back
M **NS** facial N postauricular branch
  BS facial
N **T** ability to raise one and both eyebrows

O *Erector Spinae (ES) - Iliocostalis, Longissimus, Spinalis*
  Part of the Intrinsic muscles of the back -
P *see the A-Z of Skeletal Muscles*

Q

R

S

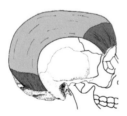
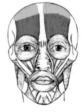

T

U

V

W

X

Y

Z

© A. L. Neill

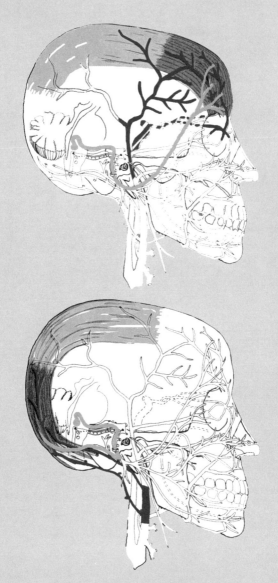

Genioglossus

BS NS

coronal

sagittal

O superior mental spine of symphysis menti (mandibular symphysis)

I ventral surface of the central mass of tongue and its mucous membrane interdigitating with intrinsic muscles of the tongue
hypoglossal membrane and the upper anterior surface of the hyoid
interdigitates with the superior pharyngeal constrictor

A protracts tongue / pokes out tongue
depression of the centre of the tongue to form a tunnel

NS C1 travelling + hypoglossal N (CN XII)

BS facial – lingual branches

T ability to poke out tongue
ability to curl up tongue into a tube/tunnel

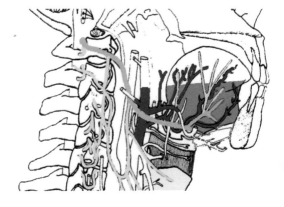

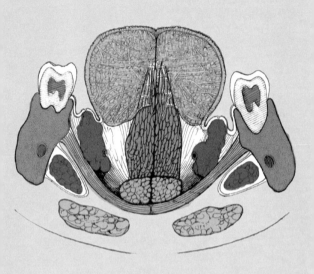

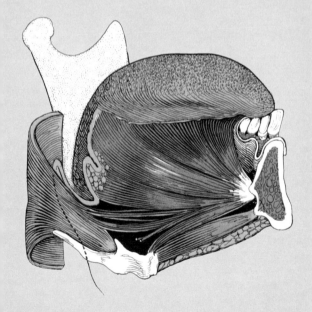

Geniohyoid

BS NS

coronal

superior

*this muscle partially determines the chin line drawing a line
b/n the Mandible and the Hyoid*

O	inferior mental spine posterior of symphysis menti (mandibular symphysis)
I	anterior surface of hyoid
A	elevation and protrusion of Hyoid
	depression of mandible (fixed hyoid)
NS	C1 travelling with hypoglossal N (CN XII)
BS	facial – mandibular branch
T	observe swallowing
	open jaw against R

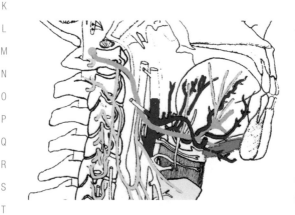

© A. L. Neill

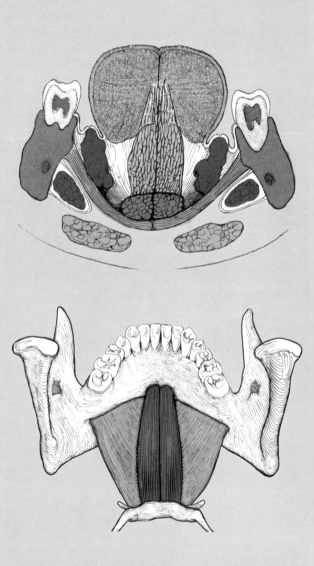

A

Hypoglossus

B

sagittal

C

O superior border + anterior surface of the hyoid bone & greater cornu

D **I** sides of the tongue, interdigitating with the intrinsic muscles of
the tongue

E **A** depresses the tongue
NS Hypoglossal N (CN XII)

F **BS** facial – lingual branches
T observe swallowing in early stages

G

H

I

J

K

L

M

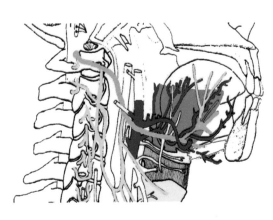

N

O

P

Q

R

S

T

U

V

W

X

Y

Z

© A. L. Neill

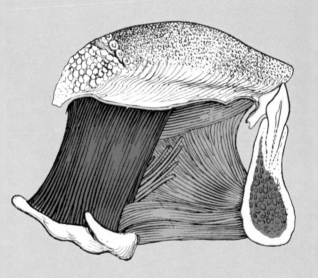

A # Iliocostalis Cervicus

B *part of ES*

C **O** angles of ribs 3-6

I TPs of cervical VBs 4-6

D **A** bilateral action - extension of the cervical spine unilateral
action - lateral flexion of the neck / cervical spine

E **NS** segmental dorsal branches of SNs

F **BS** segmental dorsal branches of the carotids

T extend neck against R and laterally flex against R

G

H

I

J

K

L

M

N

O

P

Q

R

S

T

U

V

W

X

Y

Z

© A. L. Neill

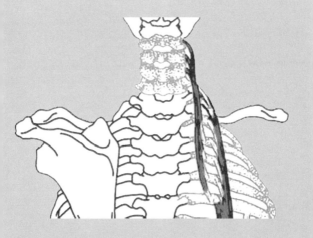

A **Incisivus Labii**

B *Inferior, Superior*

C *Upper and lower parts of the one muscle helping Orbicularis Oris to protrude lips from above and below*

D

E *Inferior*

F **O**   inferior border of mandible, lateral to mentalis, near eminence of the lateral incisor (tooth)

G **I**   into orbicularis oris + fascia at the corner of the mouth

A   protrudes lower lip

H **NS**   facial N (CN VII) inferior buccal branches

BS   facial – labial branches

I **T**   ability to protrude lips

J *Superior*

K **O**   incisive fossa of maxilla superior to the lateral incisor (tooth)

I   into orbicularis oris + levator anguli oris fascia at the corner of the mouth

L

A   protrudes upper lip

M **NS**   facial N (CN VII) superior buccal branches

BS   facial – labial branches

N **T**   ability to protrude lips

O *Note: these muscles are often missed as they lie deep to other facial muscles, and may cause imbalance or crookedness if neglected in surgery / injection procedures performed in this region*

P

Q *Inferior Lingualis see Linguali muscles*

R

S

T

U

V

W

X

Y

Z

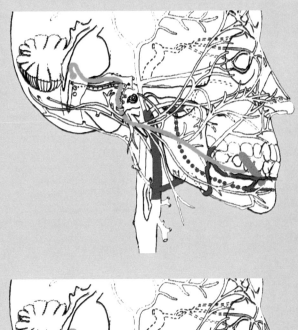

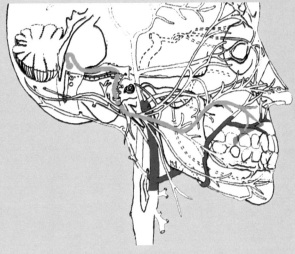

A
Inferior Oblique

B
part of the extrinsic muscles of the eye

C | **O** | orbital surface (maxilla) lateral to nasolacrimal groove

D | **I** | sclera in the back lower outer quadrant behind the equator of the eyeball b/n Inf. and Lat. Recti

E | **A** | with eye adducted - moves eyeball up with eyeball abducted - moves eyeball laterally i.e. UP & OUT

F | **NS** | oculomotor N (CN III)
| **BS** | infraorbital

G | **T** | test eye movements (note: works in conjunction with other eye muscles)

H

Inferior Pharyngeal Constrictor see Pharyngeal Constrictors

I
Inferior Rectus

J
part of the extrinsic muscles of the eye

K | **O** | inferior surface of common annular ring

L | **I** | anteroinferior surface of sclera in front of the equator of the eyeball
| **A** | with eye adducted - moves eyeball laterally with eyeball to the front -

M | moves eyeball downwards i.e. DOWN & OUT

| **NS** | oculomotor N (CN III)

N | **BS** | infraorbital, ophthalmic

| **T** | test eye movements (note: works in conjunction with other

O | eye muscles)

P

Q

R

S

T

U

V

W

X

Y

Z

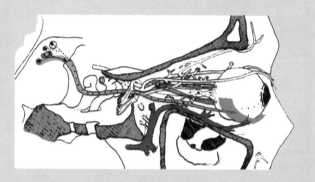

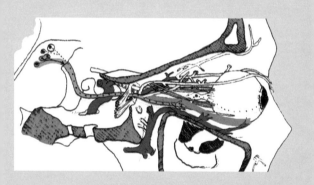

Interspinalis Cervicus

(pictured below)

(note: thoracic and lumbar regions not discussed)

O	cervical SP of C3-7
I	SP of the immediate VB above
A	draws adjacent VBs together extending the cervical VC
NS	segmental – dorsal branches of relative SNs (C1-T1)
BS	cervical – branches of the internal carotid
T	ability to extend neck / maintain upright neck position

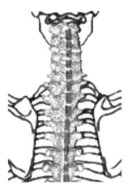

Intertransversarii Cervicus

(note: thoracic and lumbar regions not discussed)

O	cervical TP of C1-T1 on the anterior & posterior surfaces
I	TP of the immediate VB above on the same surface
A	draws adjacent VBs together extending the cervical VC
NS	segmental – ventral branches of relative SNs
BS	cervical – branches of the internal carotid
T	ability to extend and rotate neck / maintain upright neck position

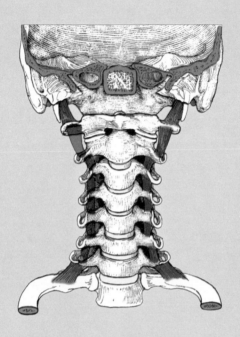

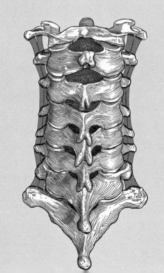

A # Lateral Cricoarytenoid

B **O** lateral aspect of cricoid arch

I muscular process of arytenoid cartilage

C **A** adductor of vocal cords -closes rima glottidis/vocal cord opening

NS recurrent laryngeal branch of vagus N (CN X)

D **BS** branches of inferior and superior thyroids

E **T** ability to open vocal cords - note this may be compromised in
stroke victims

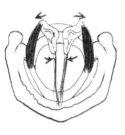

L

© A. L. Neill

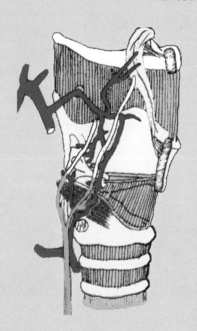

A
Lateral Pterygoid

B *part of the muscles of Mastication*

C **O** superior head - infratemporal crest of sphenoid
inferior head - lateral surface of lateral pterygoid plate of sphenoid
D **I** intra-articular cartilage of temporomandibular joint
pterygoid fovea inferior to the condyloid process of the mandible
E **A** opens jaw via depressing and protracting mandible
pulls the intra-articular cartilage of the TMJ forward
F moves mandible from side to side
G **NS** N to lateral pterygoid from trigeminal N mandibular division (CN V)
BS maxillary and its branches
H **T** open jaw against resistance

I

J

K

L

M

N

Lateral Rectus
O
part of the intrinsic muscles of the eye

P **O** inferior surface of common annular ring
Q **I** anteroinferior surface of sclera in front of the equator of the eyeball
A with eye adducted - moves eyeball laterally
R **NS** abducens N (CN VI)
BS infraorbital, ophthalmic
S **T** test eye movements (note works in conjunction with other
eye muscles)
T

U

V

W

X

Y

Z

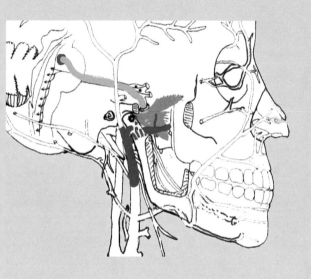

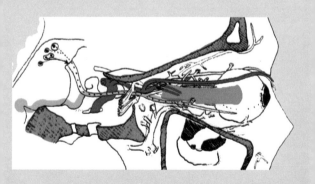

Levator Anguli Oris (Caninus)

O below the infraorbital foramen / canine fossa (maxilla)

I outer edge upper lip & modiolus interdigitating with other facial muscles and nasolabial fold

A elevates the angle of the mouth / smiling muscle

NS facial N (CN VII) buccal branches

BS facial, infraorbital

T ability to smile

Levator Labii Superioris

O infraorbital margin (maxilla and zygoma)

I upper lip interdigitating with other facial muscles

A elevates and everts the upper lip / "curling the lip"

NS facial N (CN VII) buccal branches

BS facial, infraorbital

T ability to smile

Levator Labii Superioris Alaeque Nasi

O frontal process of maxilla

I upper lip interdigitating with other facial muscles greater alar cartilages and skin of the nose

A elevates and everts the upper lip / "curling the lip" dilates nares and moves edge of nose out and up

NS facial N (CN VII) buccal branches

BS facial, infraorbital

T ability to sneer (often works unilaterally)

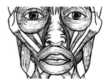

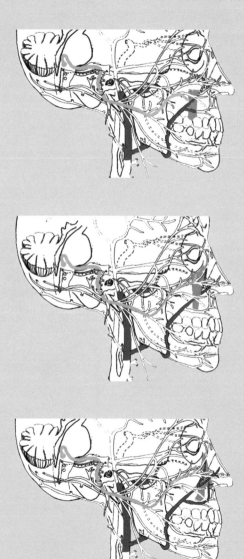

Levator Palpebrae Superioris

O inferior aspect of the lesser wing of sphenoid, superior to the optic canal

I superior tarsal plate and skin of upper eyelid

A elevates eyelid

NS oculomotor N (CN III) superior division

BS ophthalmic, supraorbital

T ability to raise eyelids "open eyes"

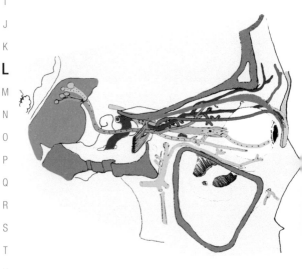

© A. L. Neill

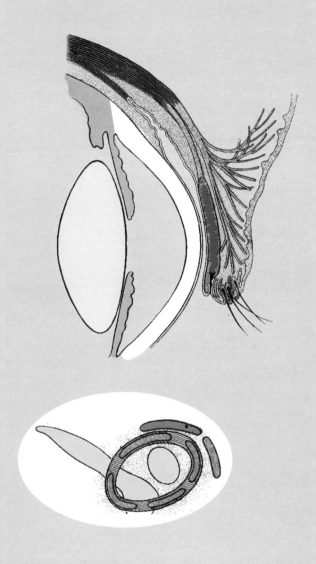

Levator Veli Palatini

O inferior surface of temporal bone - petrous part

rim of auditory tube

upper part of carotid sheath

I palatine aponeurosis

soft palate

interdigitates with its opposite and palatopharnygeus muscle and the uvulae muscularis

A vagus N (CN X) pharyngeal branch

accessory N (CN XI)

NS vagus N (CN X) pharyngeal branch accessory N (CN XI)

BS facial, maxillary ± ascending pharyngeal

T poorly functioning in snoring (like a slack "sling" flopping against the air)

may be affected in stroke victims – inability to close off the asopharynx when drinking so that fluids come out of the nose

also responsible for the yawing reflex to help open the auditory tubes when flying

Synergist

Tensor Veli Palatini

altering the shape of the Pharynx & closing the nasopharynx **T**

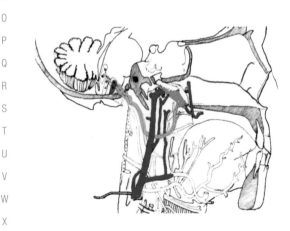

© A. L. Neill

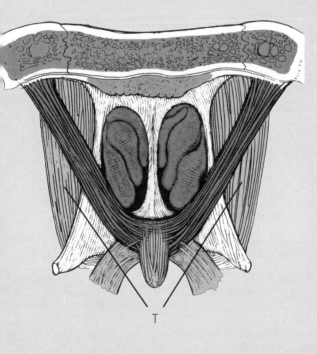

T

A

Linguali Muscles

B   *Intrinsic muscles of the Tongue – Inferior, Superior,*
C   *Transverse & Vertical*

Inferior Linguali

D

O lingual root / root of the tongue
E   body of the hyoid
I   apex of the tongue
F   **A** depresses apex and shortens tongue

G

Superior Linguali

H

O submucosa of the epiglottis
I   median fibrous septum
I   apex and margins of the tongue
J   **A** raises apex and shortens tongue

K

Transverse Linguali

L   O median fibrous septum
I   margins of the tongue
M   palatoglossus and palatoglossal arch
A narrows and elongates tongue
N

Vertical Linguali

O

O/I top to bottom of tongue at the sides (runs dorsoventrally)
P   **A** flattens and widens tongue

Q

NS hypoglossal N (CN XII)
R   **BS** lingual and branches
T   as a group test the mobility of tongue and speech clarity, ability to
S   swallow and masticate effectively

T

U

V

W

X

Y

Z

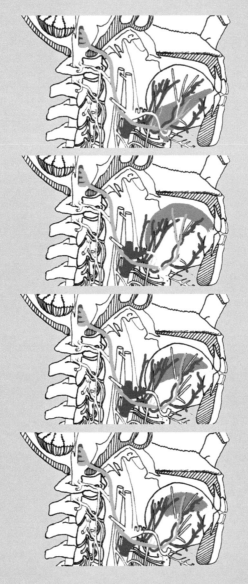

A # Longissimus Capitus

B *part of ES*

C **O** TP of T1-5
I mastoid process (temporalis)
D **A** extension and rotation of the head
NS segmental spinal roots generally the dorsal branches (C1-2)
E **BS** segmental dorsal branches of the ascending cervical BVs
F **T** ability to extend head and laterally flex head

G # Longissimus Cervicis

H *part of ES*

I **O** TP of T1-5
I TP of C2-6
J **A** extension and rotation of the neck
NS segmental spinal roots generally the dorsal branches (C1-T1)
K **BS** segmental dorsal branches of the ascending cervical BVs,
T to rotate head and neck and laterally flex

L

M

N

O

P

Q

R

S

T

U

V

W

X

Y

Z

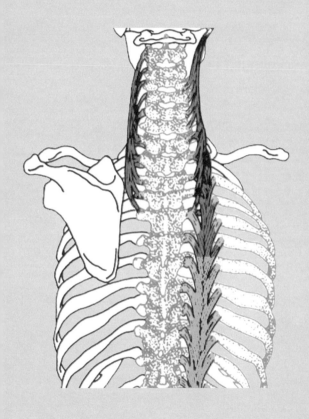

Longus Capitus

O TP of C3-7

I anterior surface of occiput

A flexion neck (bilateral action)

rotation of neck (unilateral action)

NS N to longus capitus (C1-C3)

BS vertebral – may be damaged in whiplash accidents

T flexion of neck against R

rotation of neck against R

Longus Colli

O TP and anterior surface of C1-T3

I anterior arch of atlas (C1)

A flexion neck (bilateral action)

rotation of neck (unilateral action)

NS N to longus colli (C1-C3)

BS vertebral – may be damaged in whiplash accidents

T flexion of neck against R

rotation of neck against R

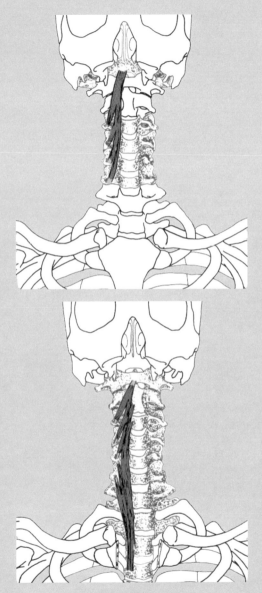

A # Masseter

B *part of the muscles of mastication*

C *has superficial and deep heads to allow for precise*
D *jaw movement*

E *transverse lateral*

O zygomatic arch (maxilla)
F **I** angle and lower ramus of the mandible, interdigitates with
medial pterygoid
G coronoid process of mandible
H **A** closes jaw
clenches teeth
I protraction and retraction of jaw
assists in side to side movement of jaw
J **NS** trigeminal N - mandibular branch (CN V$_3$)
K **BS** maxillary, facial, transverse facial
T to clench teeth and move jaw in and out

L

M

N

O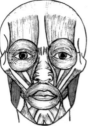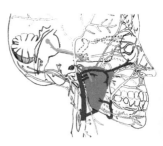

P

Q

R

S

T

U

V

W

X

Y

Z

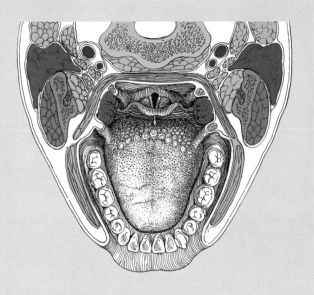

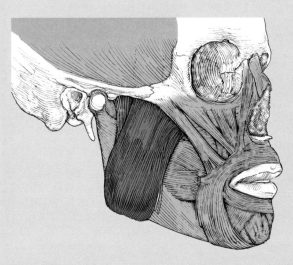

Medial Pterygoid

part of the muscles of Mastication

O medial surface of lateral pterygoid plate of sphenoid
palatine bones, maxilla

I medial surface of the angle of the mandible

A closes jaw / mandible
moves mandible back and clenches teeth
assists in side to side action of the mandible

NS trigeminal N mandibular division (CN V)

BS maxillary and its branches

T ability to clench teeth and pull jaw back

Medial Rectus

part of the extrinsic muscles of the eye

O medial surface of common annular ring

I medial surface of sclera in front of the equator of the eyeball

A moves eyeball medially - adduction ie CROSS EYED IF BOTH
CONTRACT AT ONCE

NS oculomotor N (CNIII) inf. division

BS infraorbital, ophthalmic

T test eye movements (note works in conjunction with other
eye muscles)
ability to "cross eyes"

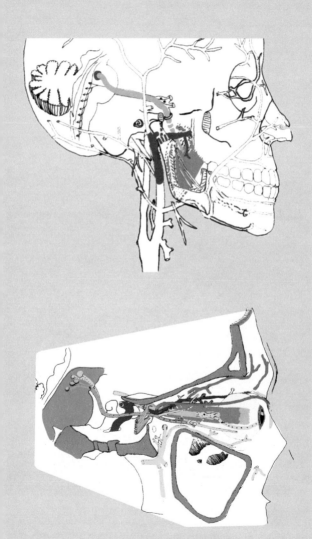

Mentalis

part of the muscles of facial expression

O   Mandible - incisive fossa
I   deep fascia of the skin of the chin
A   protrudes lips
      raises bottom lip
NS   facial N - mandibular branch (CN VII)
BS   facial - mandibular branch, inferior alveolar
T   to lift up and protrude bottom lip

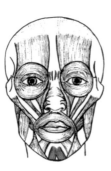

Middle Pharyngeal Constrictor see Pharyngeal Constrictors

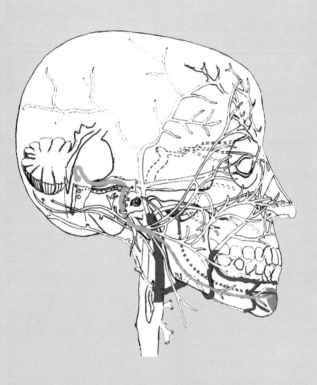

Multifidus Cervicis

part of deep spinal muscle layer

Actually multifidi is a series of small muscles responsible collectively for maintaining the cervical spine in an erect position and supporting the head. Often the source of neck pain.

O articular processes (zygapophyseal) of C1-T4

I SP of 2-3 VB above

A extension and rotation of the VC
stability of the VC

NS segmental spinal roots generally the dorsal branches (C1-T4)

BS segmental dorsal branches of the ascending cervical BVs,

T to maintain an erect and correctly postured head and neck
mobilization of this region is facilitated by these deep muscles

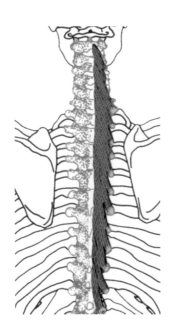

© A. L. Neill

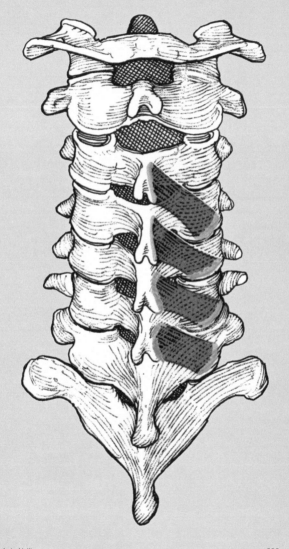

A
Mylohyoid

B
part of the muscles of the floor of the mouth determining
C
the chinline - involved in preparation of food for swallowing

D
sagittal superior

E **0** mylohyoid line (mandible)

I posterior fibres - anterior surface of hyoid

F ant. & middle fibres - decussate along median fibrous raphe
from mandibular symphysis to the hyoid

G **A** elevation ofhyoid

elevation of the floor of the mouth

H depression of mandible

NS inferior alveolar branch of trigeminal N (CNV 3rd division)

I **BS** facial – submental branch, lingual – sublingual branch,

T observe swallowing – elevation of the floor of the mouth

J

K **1** Digastricus

L **2** Tongue

M **3** Thyrohyoid

4 Geniohyoid

N

O

P

Q

R

S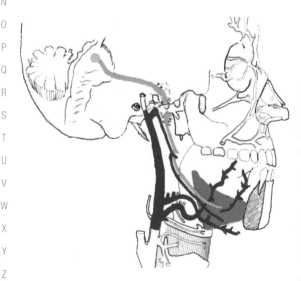

T

U

V

W

X

Y

Z

© A. L. Neill

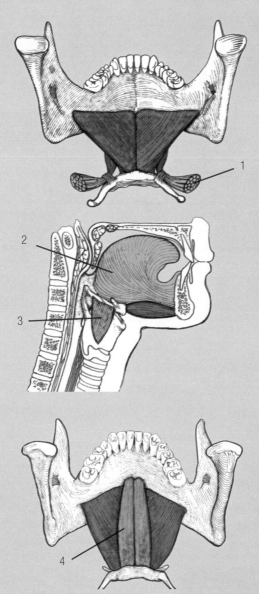

A **Nasalis**
B **Compressor Naris**
C **Dilator Naris**

D *complex pair of muscles which pull the nostrils down and*
E *flatten them, opening and closing them*

F **O** frontal process of maxilla interdigitating with procerus and
depressor septi

G **I** nasal aponeurosis (which connects it to its opposite side)
cartilaginous ala nasi

H **A** dilation and compression of nostrils in forced respiration
NS superior buccal branches of facial N (CN VII)

I **BS** facial and infraorbital branches
T no real test, observation in situations of respiratory stress

J

K

L

M

N

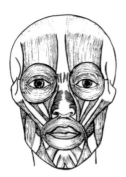

O

P

Q

R

S

T

U

V

W

X

Y

Oblique Arytenoid see Arytenoids and Aryepiglotticus

Z

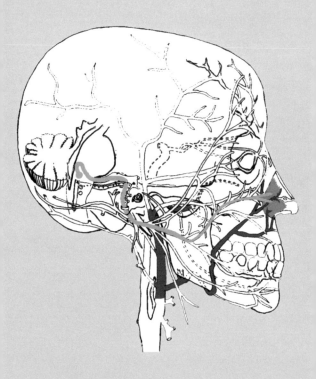

Obliquuis Capitus Inferior (i)

O   SP of C2 axis

I   TP of C1 atlas

A   rotates head at the Atlanto-axial joint

NS   suboccipital N (C2) and dorsal rami of C1-2

BS   vertebral

T   ability to rotate head ±R

Obliquuis Capitus Superior (s)

O   TP of C1 atlas

I   base of skull (occiput) lateral to the inferior nuchal line

A   extends head (bilateral)

      lateral flexion of head (unilateral)

NS   suboccipital N (C2) and dorsal rami of C1-2

BS   ascending cervical

T   ability to flex head ± R

Occipitalis see Occipito-Frontalis = Epicranius

© A. L. Neill

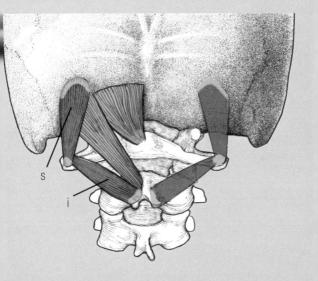

s

i

Omohyoid

part of the muscles of the Hyoid (anterior neck) two
muscular bellies inferior / superior

O   inferior – upper border of scapula inner side (lingular) of
jaw (mandible)

superior – intermediate tendon (attached to 1st rib and clavicle)

I   the inferior belly slides through a sling of deep fascia intermediate
tendon to become the superior belly and attach to the lower border
of hyoid

A   lower the raised Hyoid (for e.g. after swallowing) lower the larynx

NS ansa cervicalis (C1-3)
BS subscapular
thyroid
T   observe movement of hyoid after swallowing

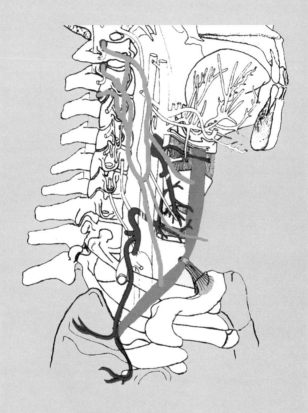

Orbicularis Oculi

part of the muscles of facial expression

O Frontalis, medial margin of maxilla, lacrimal bone

I inserts into deep fascia of the orbit on all sides lateral palpebral raphe

A tight closure of eyelids p = palpebral part
and closure of eyebrows o = orbital part
"screwing up eyes"
blinking
drainage of tear ducts

NS facial N (CN VII) temporal and zygomatic branches

BS zygomatico-orbital, palpebral branches of ophthalmic and lacrimal

T ability to "screw up eyes and eyebrows" on command against R

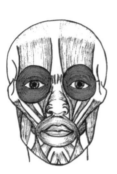

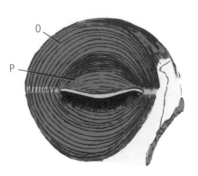

O

P

© A. L. Neill

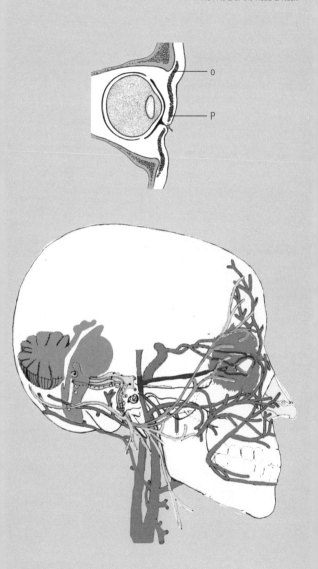

O

P

Orbicularis Oris

part of the muscles of facial expression

O Maxilla, mandible and modiolus at the angle of the mouth
I deep fascia of skin and muscles around the mouth interdigitating with surrounding muscles decussation with opposite side at the modiolus of the lips
A tight closure (deep fibres), pursing & protrusion of lips (superficial fibres) assists in the actions of other muscles here
NS facial N (CN VII)
BS facial, inferior alveolar branches
T ability to protrude lips and close mouth against R

Note: other muscles act in synergy in a lot of these actions

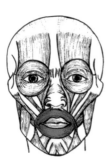

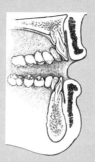

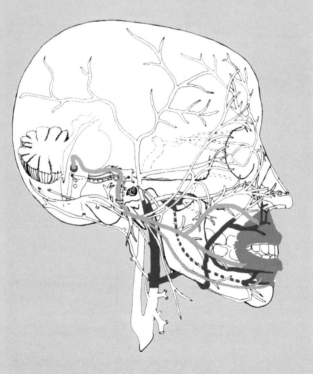

Palatoglossus

part of the Palatine Arch - palatoglossal = anterior pillar (G)

O palatine aponeurosis
I posterolateral surface of the tongue / interdigitates with its opposite and lateral lingulais
A raises the posterior of the tongue
closes oropharyngeal isthmus
initiates swallowing
NS vagus N (CN X)
BS maxillary, greater palatine branch
T ability to swallow

Palatopharyngeus

part of the Palatine Arch - palatopharyngeal = posterior pillar (P)

O palatine aponeurosis
posterior margin of the hard palate
interdigitates with its opposite,
Levator veli palatini, salpingopharyngeus and stylopharyngeus
I upper posterior border of thyroid cartilage
interdigitates with other side and with pharyngeal constrictors
A continues swallowing, raises and protracts pharynx,
closes nasopharyngeal isthmus
NS vagus N (CN X) pharyngeal branch
BS facial, maxillary, pharyngeal, palatine branches
T working together these muscles are needed to coordinate swallowing

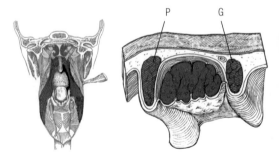

P   G

© A. L. Neill

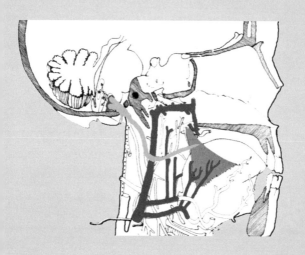

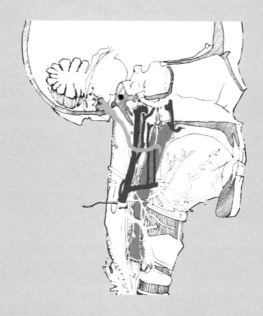

Pharyngeal Constrictors

These are circular skeletal muscles which act to coordinate swallowing before it becomes completely reflexive.

Inferior Pharyngeal Constrictor

O/I Cricopharyngeal part - lateral aspect of cricoid cartilage
Thyropharyngeus part - oblique line of thyroid cartilage connecting fibrous tissue b/n the two cartilages - fibrous cricothyroid arch

A Cricopharyngeal part acts as an upper sphincter in the oesophagus

BS thyroid arteries

Middle Pharyngeal Constrictor

O/I Anterior - lower 1/3 of the stylohyoid ligament lesser and greater cornu of the hyoid
Posterior - posterior median pharyngeal raphe interdigitates with the other constrictors

A commencement of peristaltic swallowing contractions

BS thyroid arteries, lingual

Superior Pharyngeal Constrictor

O/I Anterior - lower 2/3 of medial pterygoid plate
Pterygomandibular raphe
Mandible - mylohyoid line

I Posterior - upper part of posterior pharyngeal raphe aponeurosis to the clivus of occiput
interdigitates with middle pharyngeal constrictor

A commencement of swallowing

BS facial maxillary lingual and pharyngeal branches

NS pharyngeal plexus with fibres from: glosso pharyngeal (CN IX) vagus N (CN X), hypoglossal N (CN XI) and sympathetic fibres

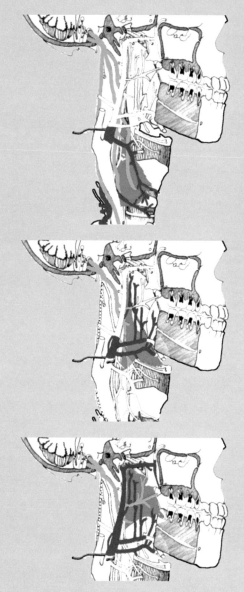

Platysma

part of the muscles of facial expression

muscle completely in the superficial fascia of the face

O superficial fascia of the upper chest

I superficial fascia of the chin and jaw up to the lower lips

interdigitates with the muscles at the modiolus of the corners of the mouth

A moves the skin from lower jaw to chest

depresses the lower lip

assists in depression of the mandible

NS facial N cervical branch (CN VII)

BS facial, inferior alveolar, laryngeal

T ability to tighten neck and jaw muscles and skin

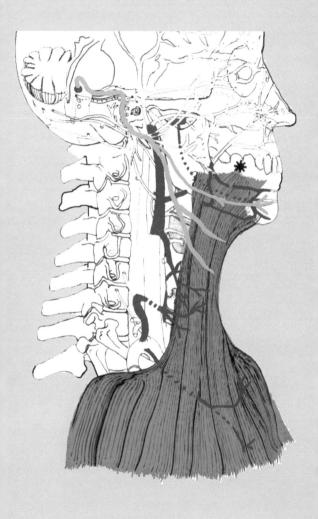

Posterior Cricoarytenoid

part of the muscles of the Larynx

O   posterior aspect of the cricoid cartilage
I   muscular process of the arytenoid cartilage
A   abducts the arytenoid cartilages opening the rima glottidis
NS   recurrent laryngeal N (branch of the vagus N = CN X)
BS   cricothyroid branches of superior and inferior thyroid arteries
T   ability to breathe

This is the only muscle which opens the normally closed rima glottidis and allows for the passage of air into the lungs - note if the recurrent laryngeal nerve is damaged it may be impossible for air to enter the trachea.

Note: the direct antagonist the CRICOARYTENOID has similar attachments but different placement causing reverse swivelling of the cartilages and closing the vocal cords.

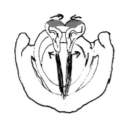

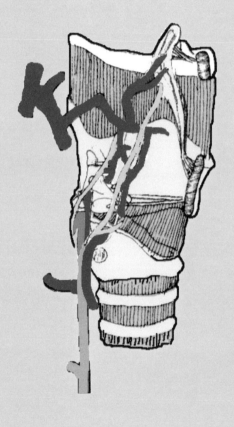

A # Procerus

B *part of the muscles of facial expression*

C **O** facial aponeurosis covering the lower part of the nose and lateral nasal cartilages

D **I** superficial fascia b/n eyebrows continuous with frontalis (epicranius)

A depresses medial end of the eyebows - frowning muscle

E **NS** facial N (CN VII) temporal branch

BS ophthalmic - supraorbital, supratrochlear branches

F **T** ability to wrinkle forehead

G

H

I

J

K

L

M

N

O

P

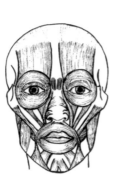

Q

R

S

T

U

V

W

X

Y

Z

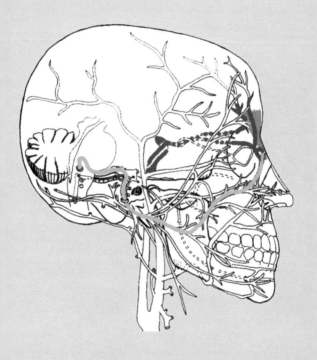

Pterygoids – Lateral, Medial

Coronal

Lateral

Posterior

Part of the muscles of Mastication.

Primary movers of the Mandible.

Lateral Pterygoid (L)

O	superior head - infratemporal crest of sphenoid
I	inferior head - lateral surface of lateral pterygoid plate of sphenoid
A	opens jaw via depressing and protracting mandible
	pulls the intra-articular cartilage of the TMJ forward
	moves mandible from side to side
NS	N to lateral pterygoid from trigeminal N mandibular division (CN V$_3$)
BS	maxillary and its branches

Medial Pterygoid (M)

O	medial surface of lateral pterygoid plate of sphenoid
	palatine bones, maxilla
I	medial surface of the angle of the mandible
A	closes jaw / mandible
	moves mandible back and clenches teeth
	assists in side to side action of the mandible
NS	trigeminal N mandibular division (CN V$_3$)
BS	maxillary and its branches
T	movements of the mandible test retraction protraction,
	side to side movements etc

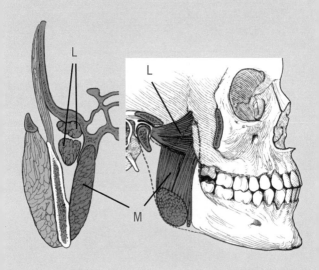

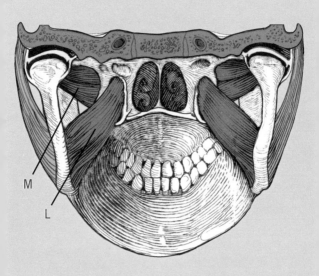

Pupillary muscles = Dilator Pupillae + Sphincter Pupillae

part of the intrinsic muscles of the eye

Dilator Pupillae

O	mesodermal stroma in the periphery of the iris
I	the iris interdigitates with the outer parts of the sphincter pupillae
A	constriction of pupil aperature for light and focus
NS	oculomotor N (CN III) - parasympathetic fibres
BS	internal carotid and ophthalmic and lacrimal branches to the eye
T	ability to adjust to light and focus

Sphincter Pupillae

O/I	collagenous connective tissue at the pupillary end of the dilator pupillae
	circumferentially around the pupil
A	constriction of pupil aperature for light and focus
NS	oculomotor N (CN III) - parasympathetic fibres
BS	internal carotid and ophthalmic branches to the eye
T	ability to adjust to light and focus

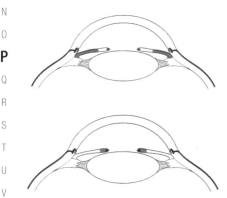

Recti muscles, part of muscles of the Eye. See Inferior Rectus, Lateral Rectus, Medial Rectus, and Superior Rectus

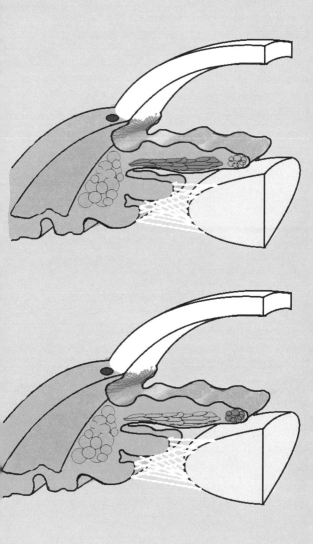

Rectus Capitus

Anterior / Lateralis / Posterior

Rectus Capitus Anterior

O   TP of atlas (C1)
I   Occiput - inferior surface of basilar part

A   flexion (head) at the atlanto-occipital joint
NS   N to rectus capitus part of CP (C2-3), suboccipital N (C1)

BS   vertebral
T   flex head against R

Rectus Capitus Lateralis

O   TP of atlas (C1)

I   Occiput - jugular process
A   lateral flexion (head) unilateral action

NS   N to rectus lateralis (C1-3) part of CP

BS   vertebral
T   laterally flex head against R

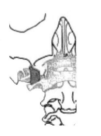

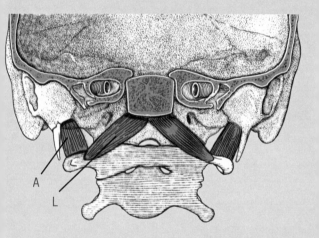

A

L

Rectus Capitus

Rectus Capitus Posterior - Major

O   SP of axis (C2))
I   Occiput - lateral to the inferior nuchal line
A   bilateral extension (head)
     unilateral ipsi-rotation - (to the same side)
NS   suboccipital N (C1)
BS   vertebral, occipital
T   extend head against R / turn head against R

Rectus Capitus Posterior - Minor

O   posterior arch of atlas (C1)
I   Occiput - medial to the inferior nuchal line
A   extension (head)
NS   suboccipital N (C1)
BS   vertebral, occipital
T   extend head against R

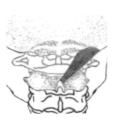

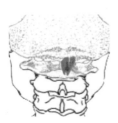

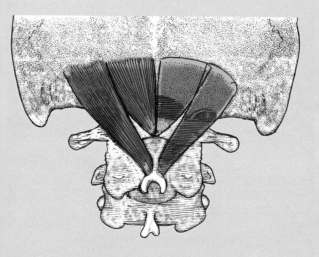

A **Risorius**

B **O**   deep fascia of the face superficial to masseter

I   skin at the angle of the mouth

C **A**   grinning (variable) - retracting the angle of the mouth

NS   facial N inferior buccal branch (CN VII)

D **BS**   facial - transverse facial branch

E

F

G

H

I

J

K

L

M

N

O

P

Q

R

S

T

U

V

W

X

Y

Z

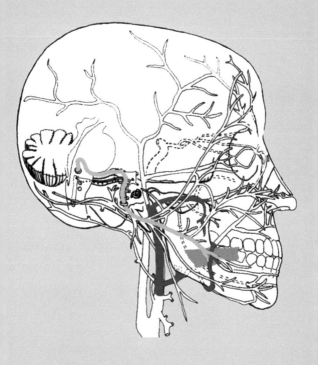

Rotatores - Longus, Brevis

part of the deepest layer of muscles of the Spine - VC
series of small muscles extending from Atlas to Sacrum
Longus completely overlays Brevis.

Has slips in the Neck - Cervicis region although not
individually named

O/I	Longus - SP to lamina of the VB 2 above
	Brevis - SP to lamina of the VB 1 above
A	bilateral - extension of the VC -neck region
	unilateral - rotation of the VC at the level of individual VBs
NS	oculomotor N (CN III)
BS	vertebral
	carotid, posterior branches of

A
B
C
D
E
F
G
H
I
J
K
L
M
N
O
P
Q
R
S
T
U
V
W
X
Y
Z

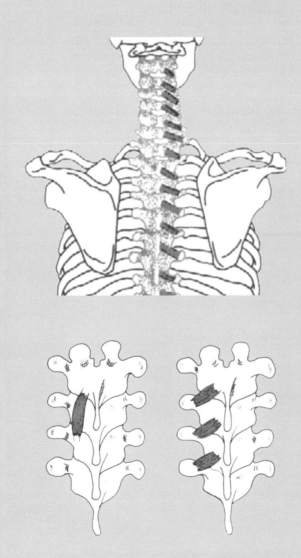

Salpingopharyngeus

part of the muscles of the anterior triangle in the neck

O   inferior surface of auditory tube

I   blends with palatopharyngeus

A   elevation of upper pharyngeal wall

        opens auditory tube in swallowing

NS   vagus N (CN X)

        accessory N (CN XI)

BS   facial, maxillary pharyngeal branches

T   ability to swallow – early stages

Note: this is the muscle which helps to equalize the pressure in the ears and why there is relief when yawning or opening the mouth in a plane

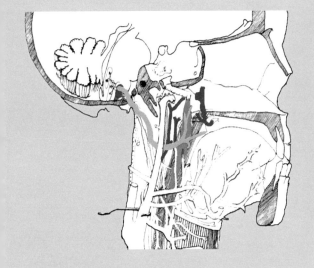

Scalenus

Anterior, Medial & Posterior (Minimus)

O   anterior   TP of C3-7

       medial   TP of C3-7

       posterior   TP of C5-7

I   anterior   anteromedial surface of rib 1

       medial   lateral to the anterior muscle rib 1

       posterior   rib 2 inferior to the clavicle

A   with fixed neck and clavicle

       elevation of the ribs in forced inspiration

       accessory muscle of inspiration

       bilateral - flexion (neck)

       unilateral - rotation & lateral flexion of the neck

NS   segmental - SNs anterior branches

       (C4-7 anterior & lateral C6-8 posterior)

       supraclavicular branches of the BP Ns (C4-8)

       N to longus colli and N to scaleni muscles

BS   superficial cervical

T   flex neck against R

       laterally flex neck against R

Note: on Scalenus Minimus - variable slip of muscle which attaches to the Suprapleural membrane (Sibson's fascia) and TP of C7 maintains the elevation of this pleura above the clavicle, often considered part of Scalenus Anterior

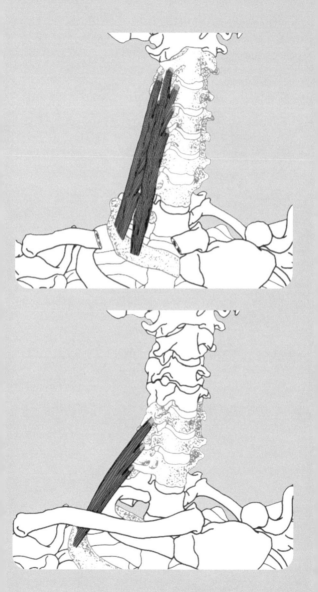

Semispinalis - Capitus, Cervicis

part of the deep muscles of the spine / neck
more lateral than Spinalis

Capitus

O   TP of C4-7
I   superior & inferior nuchal lines (Occiput)
A   bilateral extension (head)
        unilateral rotation (head)
NS suboccipital N - dorsal rami (C1)

Cervicis

O   TP of T1-6
I   SP of C1-5
A   bilateral extension (neck)
        unilateral rotation (head)
NS dorsal rami of the segmental SNs (C2-T5)
BS segmental branches from local BVs
T   ability to extend and rotate neck

Soft Palate Muscles – Musculus Uvulae, Palatoglossus, Levator &
Tensor Veli Palatini

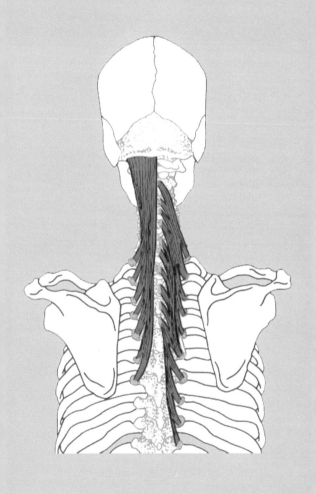

Splenius - Capitus, Cervicis

superficial to spinalis*

Capitus

O SP and supraspinous ligaments of T1-3

I lateral superior nuchal lines (occiput)
mastoid process (temporal bone)

A bilateral hyperextension, extension (head and neck)
stabilization (head)
unilateral rotation (head and neck)

NS dorsal branches of SN - dorsal rami (C1-4)
suboccipital N, greater occipital N (C1-4)

Cervicis

O ligamentum nuchae and TP of C1-3

I SP and interspinous ligaments of T1-4

A bilateral extension, hyperextension (neck and upper VC)
unilateral stabilization (neck)

NS dorsal rami of the segmental SNs (C3-8)

BS branches of the internal carotids

T neck movements

*See the A-Z of Skeletal Muscles

A
B
C
D
E
F
G
H
I
J
K
L
M
N
O
P
Q
R
S
T
U
V
W
X
Y
Z

© A. L. Neill

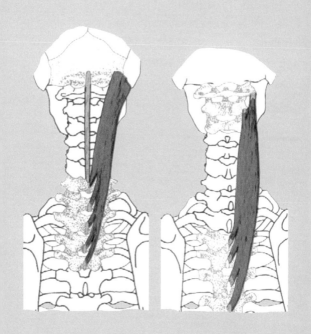

Stapedius S

O posterior wall of the inner ear

I neck of stapes

A dampens down the ossicle chain to reduce vibrations

NS facial N (CN VII) inner ear branch

BS internal carotid, maxillary, facial, middle meningeal branches

Tensor Tympani T

O cartilaginous and boney margins of the auditory tube greater wing of the sphenoid

I handle of the malleus

A pulls the Malleus medially and tenses the "ear drum"

NS N to medial pterygoid (from mandibular division of trigeminal N (CN V_3))

BS middle meningeal of mandibular pharyngeal, internal carotid branches

T involved in control of hearing adjustment to sound levels

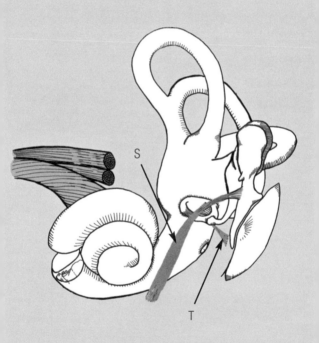

S

T

A **Sternocleidomastoid**

B **O** Manubrium (breastbone)
anterior surface of medial 1/3 of the clavicle
C **I** mastoid process (temporal bone)
anterior 1/3 of superior nuchal line
D **A** bilateral flexion (head and neck)
unilateral rotation (head and neck)
E
NS accessory N (CN XI)
F N to sternocleidomastoid (ventral rami of SNs C1-2)
BS superficial cervical
G **T** turn head against R
flex head against R

H

I

J

K

L

M

N

O

P

Q

R

S

T

U

V

W

X

Y

Z

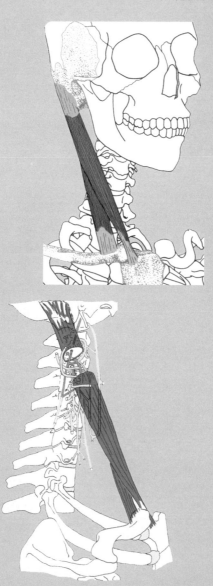

Sternohyoid

part of the muscles of the Hyoid (anterior neck)

O   posterior surface of clavicle and manubrium
I   inferior border of hyoid
A   depress the hyoid (for swallowing)
NS   ansa cervicalis (C1-3)
BS   thyroid
T   observe movement of hyoid with swallowing

Sternothyroid

part of the muscles of the anterior triangle in the neck

O   posterior surface of manubrium and 1st costal cartilage
I   oblique lines of the laminae of the thyroid cartilage
A   depress the hyoid and larynx (for swallowing)
NS   ansa cervicalis (C1-3)
BS   thyroid
T   observe movement of hyoid with swallowing

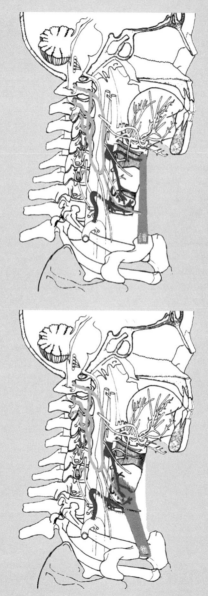

A **Styloglossus**

B *part of the Stylo-muscles - using this process for strong Muscle*

C *lateral, sagittal*

D attachment and to lift the floor of the mouth
muscles of the floor of the mouth / tongue

O apex of styloid process (sphenoid)
stylomandibular ligament
I superolateral sides of the tongue
decussating with hypoglossus
A retracts and elevates tongue
NS hypoglossal N (CN XII)
BS facial, lingual
T ability to initiate swallowing

1 Styloglossus

2 Digastricus
a - ant. belly
p. - post. belly

3 Stylohyoid

4 Fibrous sling

5 Tongue

S

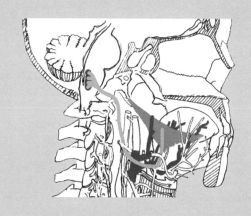

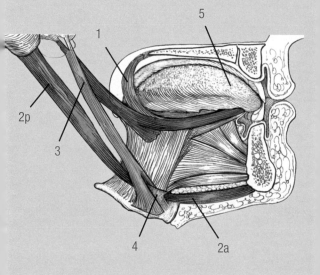

2p

2a

1

3

4

5

Stylohyoid

part of the muscles of the anterior triangle in the neck

Oblique

O   base of styloid process (sphenoid)
I   posterior surface of the hyoid to the greater cornu
A   elevate and retract the hyoid and larynx (for swallowing)
NS facial N (CN VII)
BS posterior auricular, occipital
T   ability to swallow

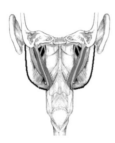

Stylopharyngeus

part of the muscles of the Pharynx

O   medial aspect of styloid process (sphenoid)
I   posteriolateral border of the laminae of the thyroid cartilage
A   elevates the hyoid and larynx (for swallowing)
NS glossopharyngeal N (CN XII)
BS thyroids, tonsillar, lingual
T   ability to swallow

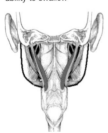

Superior Lingualis see Linguali muscles/Intrinsic muscles of the Tongue

© A. L. Neill

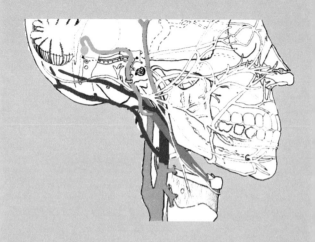

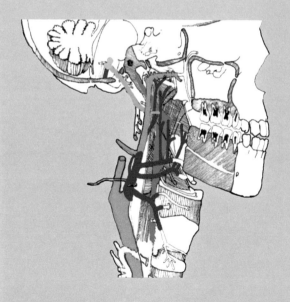

Superior Oblique

O lesser wing of sphenoid superomedial to tendinous ring

I through the trochlea/fibrocartilagenous loop to the sclera behind the equator

A depresses eye in adduction
medially rotates eye in abduction

NS trochlear N (CN IV)

BS ophthalmic

T test eye movements (note works in conjunction with other eye muscles)

Superior Pharyngeal Constrictor see Pharyngeal Constrictors

Superior Rectus

O superior tendinous ring

I superior scleral equator

A elevates eye
medially rotates eye in adduction

NS oculomotor N (CN III)

BS ophthalmic

T test eye movements
(Note: works in conjunction with other eye muscles)

A
B
C
D
E
F
G
H
I
J
K
L
M
N
O
P
Q
R
S
T
U
V
W
X
Y
Z

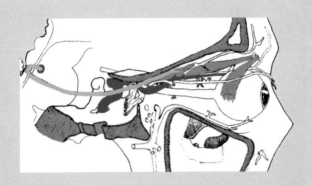

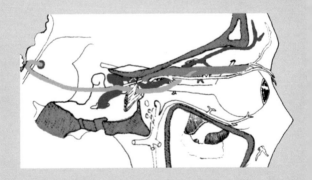

A

Temporalis

B **O** temporal fossa of the frontal, parietal and temporal bones
I coronoid process and ramus (mandible)
C **A** closes jaw
retracts mandible
D clenches teeth
E **NS** mandibular division of trigeminal N (CNV)
BS maxillary
F middle & superior temporals
T test strength of closed jaw or close against R (with care)
G

Temporoparietalis

H
O deep to temporalis, aponeurosis above auricularis
I **I** galeal aponeurosis (b/n frontalis and occipitals)
A fixes galeal aponeurosis
J **NS** facial N (CN VII)
BS maxillary
K middle & superior temporals
L **T** test strength of closed jaw or close against R (with care)

M

Tensor Tympani see Stapedius
N

O

P

Q

R

S

T

U

V

W

X

Y

Z

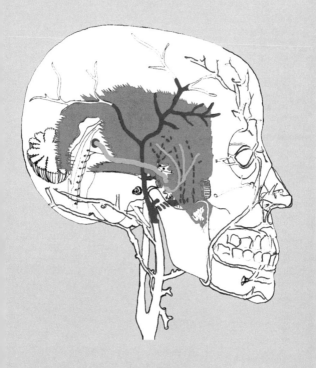

Tensor Veli Palatini

Lateral, Posterior

O scaphoid fossa (sphenoid)
rim of auditory tube (4)
spine of sphenoid

I palatine aponeurosis, crest and osseous surface
via a pulley through the pterygoid hamulus (1) of the sphenoid
soft palate
interdigitates with opposite side and uvulae muscularis (2)

A elevates soft palate, closing off nasopharynx from oropharynx -

NS N to Medial Pterygoid from mandibular division of trigeminal N(CN V)

BS facial, maxillary ± ascending pharyngeal

T poorly functioning in snoring
often affected in stroke where fluids are directed out of the nose

Synergist - **Levator Veli Palatini** which acts to support the elevation of the Pharynx area

Note: the posterior structures including the auditory tube and LVP have been removed to show the route of the muscle – and the ligamentous supports for the muscle

1 Hamulus

2 Uvulae Muscularis

3 Levator Veli Palatini

4 Auditory tube

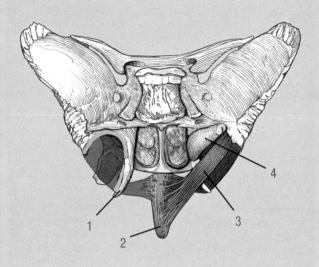

1

2

3

4

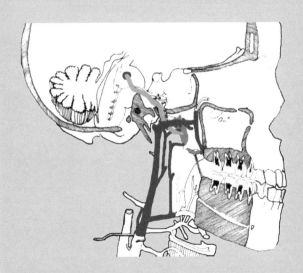

Thyroarytenoid - 1

part of the muscles of the larynx
sagittal

O   inferior surface of thyroid cartilage
       cricothyroid ligament
I   vocal processes of the arytenoid cartilages
A   relaxes the vocal folds by protracting the arytenoid cartilages

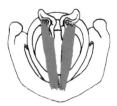

Thyroepiglotticus - 2

O   lower posterior surface of thyroid cartilage
I   epiglottic fold and margin
A   closes additus to the larynx

NS vagus N (CN X) recurrent laryngeal branch
BS thyroids pharyngeal branches
T   ability to change voice tone

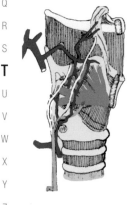

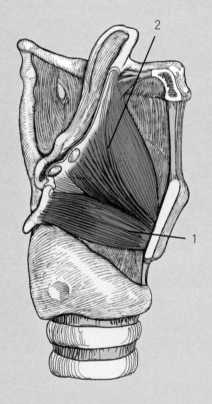

A # **Thyrohyoid**

B *part of the muscles of the anterior triangle in the neck*

C **O** oblique lines of the laminae of the thyroid cartilage
I Hyoid - cornu and body
D **A** depresses & elevates the larynx
NS C1 with hypoglossal N (CN XII)
E **BS** thyroid
T observe movement of hyoid with swallowing
F

G *Transverse Arytenoid see Arytenoids*

H
Transverse Lingualis see Linguali muscles/Intrinsic muscles of the
I *Tongue*

J *Vertical Lingualis see Linguali muscles/Intrinsic muscles of the Tongue*

K

L

M

N

O

P

Q

R

S

T

U

V

W

X

Y

Z

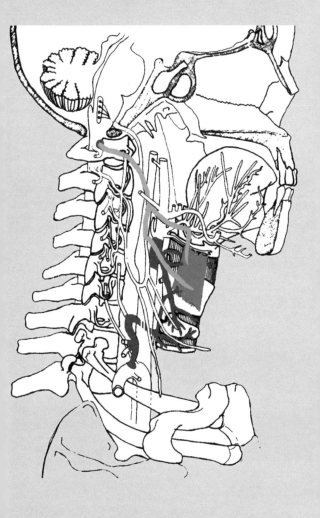

A **Uvulae Muscularis** aka Muscularis Uvulae

B *Part of the muscles of the pharynx*

C *posterior*

D *sagittal*

E **O** posterior border of hard palate
palatine aponeurosis

F **I** uvular mucosa

A elevation and retraction of the uvula

G **NS** pharyngeal branch of vagus N (CNX) and accessory N (CNXI)

BS maxillary -greater palatine branch

H **T** say AHHH and watch uvula

I 1 Hyoid bone

J 2 Superior pharyngeal constrictor

K 3 Tongue

L 4 Oropharynx

M 5 Levator veli palatini

6 Auditory tube

N

O

P

Q

R

S

T

U

V

W

X

Y

Z

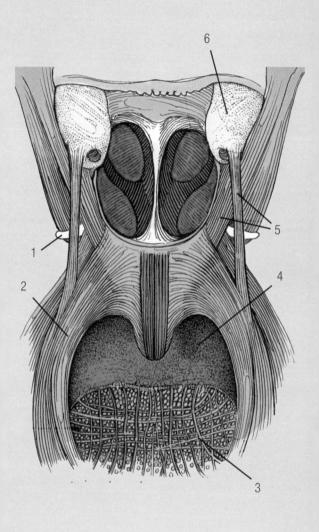

A **Vocalis**

B *part of the muscles of phonation (voice production)*

C *Superior*

D Moves the arytenoid cartilages and changes the tension on the vocal cords

E **O** orbital surface (maxilla) inferior surface of thyroid cartilage

F cricothyroid ligament

I vocal processes of the arytenoid cartilages

G **A** relaxes the vocal folds by protracting the arytenoid cartilages

NS vagus N (CN X) recurrent laryngeal branch

H **BS** thyroids pharyngeal branches

I **T** ability to change voice tone

J 1 Arytenoid cartilage

K 2 Vocal cord

L 3 Thyroarytenoid

4 Thyroid cartilage

M

N

O

P

Q

R

S

T

U

V

W

X

Y

Z

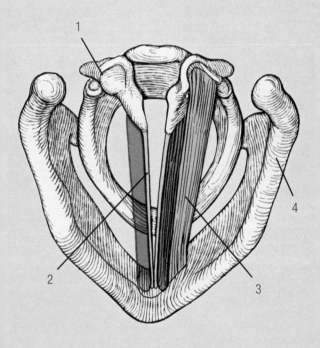

Zygomaticus – Major, Minor

part of muscles of facial expression

Zygomaticus Major

O   Zygoma - cheekbone
I   deep fascia at the angle of the mouth (modiolus)

A   draws mouth back smiling/laughing
NS facial N (CN VII)

BS facial
T   smile

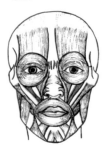

Zygomaticus Minor

O   Zygoma - cheekbone
     deep fascia of the upper lip

A   maintains nasolabial furrow - philtum
     everts upper lip

NS recurrent laryngeal N
BS facial

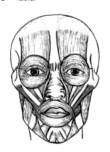

Often lost in cosmetic surgery i.e. no skin crease from nose to lips.

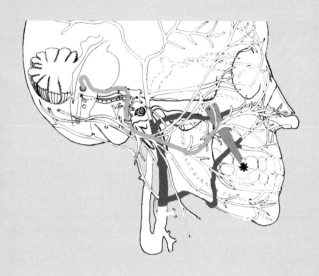

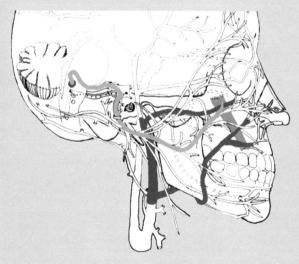